Home-Prepared Dog and Cat Diets

D1235973

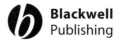
Blackwell
Publishing

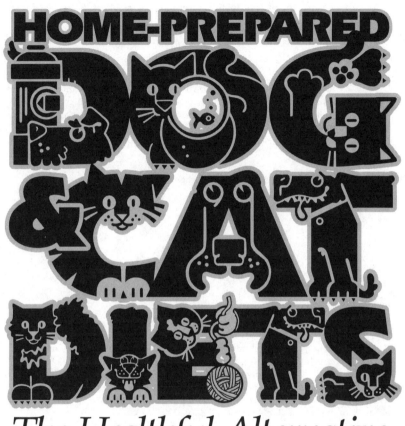

HOME-PREPARED DOG & CAT DIETS

The Healthful Alternative

Donald R. Strombeck, DVM, PhD

Disclaimer: Every effort has been made to ensure that the information in this book is accurate; however, errors may be present. The author and publisher assume no responsibility for and make no warranty with respect to results obtained from the procedures, treatments, recipes, or dosages used, nor shall the author or publisher be held liable for any misstatements or errors that may have been obtained by any person or organization using this book.

Donald R. Strombeck, Dvm, PHD, is Professor Emeritus, University of California, Davis, School of Veterinary Medicine, as well as an honorary member of the College of Veterinary Internal Medicine. He is widely published and has received numerous awards, including the Ralston Purina Award for research excellence for his work in gastroenterology. Dr. Strombeck practiced as a clinician in small animal medicine for over 40 years.

Design by Robert Mickey Hager, Hager Design

© 1999 Iowa State University Press
All rights reserved

Blackwell Publishing Professional
2121 State Avenue, Ames, Iowa 50014

Orders: 1-800-862-6657
Office: 1-515-292-0140
Fax: 1-515-292-3348
Web site: www.blackwellprofessional.com

Authorization to photocopy items for internal or personal use, or the internal or personal use of specific clients, is granted by Blackwell Publishing, provided that the base fee of $.10 per copy is paid directly to the Copyright Clearance Center, 222 Rosewood Drive, Danvers, MA 01923. For those organizations that have have been granted a photocopy license by CCC, a separate system of payments has been arranged. The fee code for users of the Transactional Reporting Service is 0-8138-2149-5/99 $.10.

Printed on acid-free paper in the United States of America

First edition, 1999

Library of Congress Cataloging-in-Publication Data
Strombeck, Donald R.
   Home-prepared dog and cat diets: the healthful alternative/Donald R. Strombeck
      p.   cm.
   Includes bibliographical references (p.   ) and index.
   ISBN 0-8138-2149-5
   1. Dogs—Food—Recipes.   2. Cats—Food—Recipes   3. Dogs—Nutrition.
   4. Cats—Nutrition   5. Dogs—Diseases—Diet therapy.   6. Cats—Diseases—Diet
   therapy.   I. Title
   Sf427.4.S77   1999
   636.7"0855—dc21   98-39308

The last digit is the print number: 9 8

To my friend and colleague, Quinton R. Rogers

CONTENTS

PREFACE

Diet is the most important consideration in a pet's care; it determines health and life expectancy. *Home-Prepared Dog and Cat Diets: The Healthful Alternative* is about foods for a long, healthy life and is also written for pets with health problems that can be managed dietarily. This handbook is unique in providing nutritional and dietary guidance not provided by veterinarians. These diets are formulated with a computer program to ensure that they are balanced and complete. The program also ensures proper modification of diets necessary for management of health problems. Nutrient content for proteins, fats, and calories is given for all diets, and mineral content is given for a number of special diets. The diets are prepared from unprocessed foods marketed for human consumption that are readily available in any large food market. Pet owners can control the quality and wholesomeness of a diet's ingredients.

No other book of this type has been published. *Home-Prepared Dog and Cat Diets: The Healthful Alternative* developed out of the author's 44-year clinical small animal medicine experience in private practice and a veterinary medical teaching hospital. This experience was with many clients who wished to prepare their pets' diets. These clients did not want to feed their pets a commercial pet food, and for many patients no commercial pet food could resolve their problems. A recipe for an owner-prepared diet was necessary.

The pet food industry convinces veterinarians and pet owners that only commercially prepared foods offer complete and balanced diets. The industry claims that medical problems will be encountered by feeding owner-prepared diets. It tells the public that feeding human foods may actually harm American companion animals whose owners have been misled to believe that they can give their animal something from their own meal, thinking that their human food will fulfill the animal's needs. The industry believes that average owners cannot prepare and feed their pets a complete and balanced diet. Unfortunately, commercially prepared diets are not always complete and balanced, and just as important they offer no choice about quality and wholesomeness, which are of utmost importance.

Before the 1960s many if not most owners prepared their pets' diets, and few nutritional problems were seen. Since then nutritional problems have been seen but mostly in animals fed commercial pet foods. Today the media provides ample instructions on nutrition. With this nutritional knowledge, pet owners have an excellent background for preparing diets to feed healthy and sick pets under guidance of a veterinarian.

PART ONE
Food Quality and Safety

CHAPTER 1
Introduction

A Human Need—Dogs and Cats

Ten thousand years ago human beings began domesticating dogs and cats and used them for herding livestock, hunting game, and controlling vermin. Their primary role today is for companionship and pleasure, with few doing any work. People who value their relationship with small animal pets recognize the need for maintaining pets' health to keep them fit. This book is about feeding pets to support a long and healthy life. How a pet is fed determines its health and life expectancy more than any other care.

Feeding Pets to Ensure a Long and Healthy Life

Adequate and balanced nutrition is necessary for all life's well-being. Inadequate nutrition produces many disease conditions and can shorten life expectancy. This book describes new aspects of nutrition and dietetics for maintaining the health of dogs and cats. It is important because it gives pet owners a choice in their animals' diets. For most dogs and cats there is little dietary choice available.

> Most of the world's companion animals depend on humans to supply their nutritional needs. In their native state, cats and dogs apparently selected nutritionally complete and balanced diets, but with domestication generally a single food is presented, which eliminates the choice animals previously exercised.[1]

3

Feeding a single food such as commercial pet food virtually eliminates any dietary choice humans can make for their pets.

Dogs and cats require a nutritionally complete and balanced diet to support normal growth of young animals and to sustain maintenance needs of adults. Pet foods are generally adequate in meeting nutritional needs, but they are not always nutritionally complete and balanced.[1] Problems sometimes develop because of nutrient deficiency or excess. Thereby, diets and eating habits can contribute to medical problems and reduced life expectancy. This concern has been voiced to the pet food industry.

> *Pets are breaking down from disease at an unprecedented rate from a variety of problems. Why are so many pets getting cancers, renal failures, hepatic diseases, multitudes of skin and coat problems? Diseases and illnesses we simply shouldn't be seeing. Illness and poor nutrition affect each other.*
>
> *With relatively large numbers of pets getting sicker and sicker, we should take a serious look at what we've been providing for them. Food is clearly not the only determinant of health, but it is one of the only health-related factors pet owners can control.[2]*

Surprisingly, "most of our prehistoric ancestors had better diets and health than we do."[3] Early humans foraged for food just like dogs and cats in earlier times. When foraging stopped, humans developed dramatic changes in one of the few signs of evolution that scientists can look at today, their skeletal structure. The changes were not due to evolution but to changes in diets and lifestyle. These changes put humanity on a path toward poorer, not better, diets. For many, the poorer diets were based on eating corn. No longer foraging and eating "more perfect" diets, the foragers-become-farmers showed degenerative diseases not found in their foraging ancestors. The foragers were much more healthy and "almost totally free of internal parasitic infections."[3] The conclusion is that "degenerative changes seen with aging develop after a lifetime of neglect, in particular, eating improper foods and getting little exercise."[3]

Diets prepared for our pets today are very different from the diet of a foraging animal. Current diets are based on cereals, similar to humans' diets when they stopped foraging. These diets are nutritionally adequate in being complete and balanced but do not ensure maximum life expectancy. A number of canine and feline medical problems significantly relate to such diets. These problems are discussed throughout this book.

Americans can easily learn enough about nutrition and dietetics to prepare a diet for a dog or cat. Owners rarely plan and prepare meals for their pets, however. They leave that to the pet food industry, which claims that only nutritional experts have competence to formulate a pet's diet.

Nutritional Education of Pet Owners

Veterinarians should educate people on feeding pets. Counseling owners on feeding is the most important client education a veterinarian can offer. This education must be more than to advise feeding a commercial pet food. A pet can be fed foods consumed by human beings.

Client education begins with instruction on feeding puppies and kittens, which establishes a pattern for lifelong pet care, an important practice of preventive health. Education on feeding should promote wellness and identify risks for preventable medical problems. A good knowledge about feeding can prevent many medical problems.

Sources of Nutritional Knowledge

Veterinarians often provide little nutritional education because the pet food industry has "taken this off their hands."[4] The industry prints and distributes feeding information for veterinarians to give clients. Pet food companies use such information to promote sales. The industry's nutritional experts educate veterinarians and veterinary students to use their products. This hasn't improved veterinarians' knowledge about nutrition. A survey of veterinarians indicated that nutrition training is inadequate in veterinary schools and quality of continuing education on nutrition is inferior.[5]

Pet owners are interested in nutrition and dietetics, which is pointed out in a book written to provide the practicing veterinarian with up-to-date information on canine nutrition and feeding management, a book that would be useful for veterinarian, pet owner, and dog:

> One need only read the health sections of major newspapers and week-ly news magazines to gauge the level of public interest in nutrition. A number of subjects have been scrutinized: food additives, preservatives, known or suspected carcinogens, dietary cholesterol and its effect on cardiovascular disease, megavitamin therapy, and dietary influence on tumor behavior to name but a few. Coupled with the public interest is a

major movement away from highly processed foods back to "natural" or basic "organic" food sources.

Some argue that the focus of attention has turned toward nutrition as a direct result of the social concerns raised over the ever-expanding world population and the projected inadequacy of food supply and delivery systems. Others see it in part as a personalization of the environmental movement. The heightened awareness of the importance of nutrition is probably also influenced by the success of modern medicine in eliminating many of the diseases which at one time were the major causes of death in the population.

Regardless of the reasons, concern about nutrition has reached an all-time high. Many people are vitally concerned about the quality of their diet and its effect on their personal and family health. It stands to reason, then, that the pet-owning public will transfer these concerns to the nutrition of their pets as well.

Over the past decade, our knowledge of canine nutrition has grown steadily. Sadly, however, only a variable amount of this information has reached the practicing veterinarian whose knowledge of canine nutrition is often not much more advanced that it was decades ago. Today we know much more about the varying dietary needs at different stages in a dog's life; about different needs for different diseases; about the relationship between diet and a dog's ability to deal with stress.

Questions from clients about nutrition at one time were simple. What kind of dog food is best? What food do you recommend? How much and how often do I feed? These questions were easily handled and required very little sophisticated knowledge of nutrition. However, as clients become more involved with their own nutrition, questions posed to veterinary practitioners become more complicated.

This changing awareness and interest affords us all a tremendous opportunity to improve client relations. Clients are seldom aware of the extent of our knowledge and skills. Very often they bring us their ill and injured pets and take them home well or healing. Many clients, however, never realize the many complicated steps that occur between admission and discharge. Much of their impression of the profession is based upon how we answer their questions. Nutritional guidance, then, is not a subject to be taken lightly. We now have the opportunity to show our clients a part of the knowledge required to be a veterinary professional. Equally important at this "teaching moment" is the chance to guide dog owners on improving the health of their animals.[6]

Home-Prepared Dog and Cat Diets: The Healthful Alternative provides unique nutritional guidance. In addition to owner-prepared recipes is information on nutritional counseling for use during client-patient visits. Pet owners must be educated that diet is essential for recovery from many medical problems; cures are not found only in drugs or surgery.

Faulty Diets and Inadequate Nutrition

Inadequate nutrition in pets can be explained two ways. Faulty diet was an acceptable explanation in the past but is seldom a reason today. Poor feeding management rather than faulty diet is believed responsible for many nutritional problems.[7] Finding the right diet solves nutritional problems. The pet food industry claims optimum nutrition and health for animals fed the correct commercial pet food. What should veterinarians advise clients on their pets' diets? "More often it means providing the dog owner with a simple framework to aid in grasping the basics of canine nutrition."[7] That means helping select the correct commercial diet. But any diet, including commercial diets, can be faulty so that faulty management is not the only cause of inadequate nutrition. The primary purpose of this book is to instruct veterinarians and clients on preparing complete and balanced diets for both healthy and sick pets.

The pet food industry discourages owners from preparing a pet's diet. It proclaims:

> Most people who have a cat or a dog do not have the degree of nutritional expertise, access to the appropriate raw materials, the time or the desire to pursue complicated preparation and cooking of food for their pets. As a consequence the manufacture of foods specially prepared for cats and dogs has developed, particularly over the last forty years, into what is now a large and sophisticated industry.[8]

> Homemade diets are now rarely fed to dogs because of the availability of good, economical proprietary foods. However, some owners still elect to feed table scraps or to manufacture their own diets. These diets are rarely consistent from day to day and may vary considerably in their protein, carbohydrate, fat and vitamin content. Foods such as potatoes, cereals, and bread, if fed in large amounts, often precipitate diarrhea. [Cereals are the main ingredient in most dog foods.] Overcooking food will reduce its digestibility and lead to dietary diarrhea, while dogs maintained on fresh meats diets often have foul smelling fluid diarrhea. In all cases establishing a normal dietary routine will relieve the signs. This may

have to be carried out in a hospitalized environment as owners often feel their dog will not eat commercial diets.[9]

Veterinarians are educated to believe that owner-prepared diets are likely to be faulty and cause medical problems. Human beings have the nutritional expertise to prepare their own diets; that same expertise can be used to feed their pets. Human beings develop nutritional problems mostly from consuming processed foods rather than ones they prepare themselves. Pet owners control dietary quality and wholesomeness when they prepare their animals' diets themselves. Control is maintained over nutritional adequacy.

Balancing a Diet

Pet owners are advised to select foods labeled "balanced" or "complete"; such diets ensure a long and healthy life. What does it mean to label a diet balanced? "A balanced diet contains optimal proportions of nutrients so that they can be utilized with maximal efficiency for a specific purpose."[7] No one knows how to precisely formulate a diet with optimal amounts of nutrients, however. The amount of any needed nutrient falls in an optimal range rather than being a specific amount. Variable individual needs under varying conditions decide a range's breadth. Errors and imprecision in nutritional methods also decide the breadth. The optimal range is broader for maintenance of an adult animal living under conditions demanding small energy consumption. The range is narrower for animals with greater needs such as during growth, breeding, and hard work or stress.

Feeding a diet deficient in one or more nutrients affects performance and ability to gain weight. Inadequacies also affect number of offspring and ability to function or withstand stress. Feeding a marginally adequate diet may result in no signs in a sedentary animal. However, with the addition of stress, that diet is nutritionally inadequate. Minimum optimal levels for nutrients usually change for different physiological functions, such as physical activity, pregnancy, lactation, and growth.

Excess of any nutrient can be toxic at certain levels. Some nutrients have a narrow range between adequacy and toxicity. Such nutrients are more likely to cause toxicity because of the way a diet is formulated or an animal is fed. Variation is also found for an animal's ability to metabolize or excrete nutrients. With such ability limited, a nutrient can become toxic because its excretion lags behind intake.

The pet food industry does not measure some important nutrients in its products. Manufacturers admit to adding excesses for some nutrients to ensure adequate levels in a product: "Loss of nutrients, particularly of vitamins, is limited because of baking or extrusion temperatures or time and sufficient supplements are added to counterbalance processing and storage losses."[8] Supplementation to remedy this estimate of loss often results in some nutrients being in excess.

Requirements for a Diet to Be Balanced and Complete

■ Pet Food Standards

What can be known about commercial pet foods that are complete or balanced? Pet food labels state whether nutrients are provided at levels required to be adequate for all life stages of an animal. This claim allows the label to describe the food as complete, perfect, scientific, or balanced. How is a diet produced so it can be labeled as balanced or complete? Manufacturers can make this claim when they formulate diets following recommendations established by the Committee of Animal Nutrition of the National Research Council (NRC) of the National Academy of Science. The NRC selects a committee to evaluate nutritional requirements and to set standards for pet foods to meet these requirements. That committee is *the* authority on estimating nutrient requirements for all life stages of a dog or cat. For many years the NRC was the only group to establish the standards for feeding dogs, cats, and other animals; all references to a diet being complete and balanced were based on the NRC standards. The pet food industry is now discarding all reference to the NRC and is establishing its own standards.

■ Industry Abandons NRC "Gold Standard"

The pet food industry created a group called the Association of American Feed Control Officials (AAFCO), which can either adopt NRC standards or establish its own, depending on the wishes of the industry. In 1974 the AAFCO adopted NRC recommendations for using feeding trials to evaluate adequacy for pet foods. Such testing was too restrictive for some sections of the industry, however. Thus, the AAFCO designed an alternate procedure for claiming nutritional adequacy for a pet food. Instead of feeding a food to evaluate its adequacy, chemical analysis was done to decide if it would meet or exceed

NRC requirements. However, nothing can be derived from chemical analysis about palatability, digestibility, and biological availability of nutrients. This lack of information on digestibility and biological availability means chemical analyses do not indicate whether a pet food can fulfill an animal's nutrient needs. The AAFCO was aware of the limitations of chemical analyses and "solved" the problem by adding "fudge" or "safety" factors that established the AAFCO's own requirements for exceeding the minimum.[1] The nutritional requirement with the added safety factor is a nutritional allowance.

The pet food industry abandoned the NRC's guidelines following the NRC's 1985 revision of *Nutrient Requirements of Dogs*. The NRC challenged and upset the industry by the revision's statement "Users are advised to obtain evidence of nutritional adequacy by direct feeding to dogs." On discarding the NRC standards the AAFCO established itself as the authority for industry to follow; the industry established its own standards. With the AAFCO establishing the "gold standard," pet food manufacturers no longer must follow NRC standards for formulating a pet food. Anyone can produce pet food merely by following the AAFCO's formulas.

In the 1985 NRC revised *Nutrient Requirements of Dogs*, nutritionists renewed the call for feeding trials to determine whether pet foods are complete and balanced. Feeding trials must be done to show that animals fed a pet food remain healthy and grow or maintain body weight, depending on their age and stage of life. What is the effect of this NRC position? "It challenges the pet food industry; 'Users are advised to obtain evidence of nutritional adequacy by direct feeding to dogs'(NRC, 1985)."[10]

That disappointed and angered the industry.

> *The response of the pet food industry to the change in the 1985 NRC report, to the all-important caveat that a simple "meets or exceeds" is unacceptable and that dog feed protocols may be mandatory, ranged from disappointment to anger. The AAFCO regulatory officials have yet to make a firm decision on this point in spite of the fact that they had two years advance notice that these changes were coming. Until they do decide, all label claim regulations will continue to use the 1974 revision as their guide.[11]*

With the AAFCO's current position, feeding trials are no longer required. (With the AAFCO setting the standard, not even the 1974 NRC revision continues as the guide.) The larger pet food companies may do some, but the smaller companies are likely to conduct no feeding trials. The AAFCO did some feeding trials on three generic pet foods. It believes that no additional trials are necessary if the manufacturer uses the formula of any of these generic foods. That poses severe limitations, however.[11]

■ The Need for Feeding Trials

Manufacturers can legitimately claim foods are balanced or complete only by feeding them with no other source of nourishment. Testing must show that the food is satisfactory for whatever claims are made. The claims include maintains weight for normal animals; is satisfactory for normal growth from weaning to maturity; and is satisfactory for female fertility, gestation, and lactation. However, the pet food industry chooses not to mandate feeding trials. It is currently solving this dilemma with the NRC by no longer following the NRC recommendations but by using its own approach that is officially sanctioned by the AAFCO.

Most likely, the pet food industry through its own committee, the AAFCO, abandoned the NRC oversight of pet food adequacy in order to avoid the costs of evaluating any diet. There are many small manufacturers of pet foods who do not conduct protocol feeding tests. Such testing costs $7000 to $10,000 per diet. Furthermore they are likely not to completely analyze a diet chemically, which costs about $2000.

Establishing Nutritional Adequacy

Diets cannot be formulated to have optimal nutrient levels based merely on results from nutritional studies such as those reported by the NRC; only feeding studies determine adequacy for any commercial pet food.[1] Many pet foods are largely based on cereals as their source of proteins. Cereals are very deficient in at least one essential amino acid, lysine. Manufacturers mix meat products with cereals so the final product has adequate amounts of lysine. It can be added by using meat and bone meal, but this product can also be deficient in lysine. The deficiency is evident in feeding trials or chemical analyses of the final product, tests that many manufacturers do not conduct. Pet foods can also be deficient in available trace minerals such as iron and copper. These minerals are usually added in the form of their salts. Copper and iron absorption and use vary according to the form used. Thus, one form may be so poorly absorbed that the diet is deficient even though the total amount may exceed NRC requirements. That may also cause the producer to add a great excess to ensure no deficiency, but the excess can also be toxic. Without analyses and feeding trials, a diet may be deficient even though it can be labeled as complete and balanced. Nutrients in a food can also be inadequate because of their interactions. Excess of one essential nutrient can induce another's deficiency. For example, the need for vitamin E increases on feeding high levels of polyunsaturated fats. High levels of calcium increase requirements for zinc and can induce zinc deficiency. Diets containing excess zinc increase the requirement for copper to prevent copper deficiency. Chemical analyses of diets do not reveal such inadequacies.

Nutritional studies such as those reported in the NRC's *Nutrient Requirements of Dogs* may not establish nutrient requirements for another reason.[1] The least amount of a nutrient such as histidine for supporting maximum growth is not enough to maintain hemoglobin concentration or to prevent cataract formation.[1] Thus, there is not merely one requirement for a nutrient. There is a whole range of requirements that depends on the need in every body system and the animal's needs for physiological performance. The minimal requirement for a growing animal is that which promotes maximal growth without regard to needs of specific tissues. To be concerned with what happens in all body tissues, it is necessary to test pet foods in feeding trials. Formulating a diet from AAFCO recommendations cannot serve that purpose. Diets cannot be formulated theoretically: any such formulation is too imprecise for meeting animals' needs.

The industry knows that diet formulation to produce complete and balanced diets is imprecise, so it employs safety factors and adds excess nutrients. Is that justified?

> *Does an intake of a nutrient in excess of the nutritional requirement promote greater health than at the requirement? When diets are prepared to contain just the minimal amount of a nutrient there is always the risk the minimum will not be achieved because of natural variation in nutrient content of foods, bioavailability of the nutrient and the individual nutrient requirement. Therefore it is potentially dangerous to formulate diets just at the minimum. On the other hand, most nutrients in excess are toxic and so a huge excess of a nutrient is generally not appropriate. Some nutrients such as methionine have a very narrow range between requirement and toxicity, others such as the B vitamins have a wide range between requirement and toxicity.[12]*

If this statement is true, the pet food industry should use NRC recommendations to formulate the best balanced and complete diet and conduct feeding trials to prove its adequacy.

Dogs and cats consumed complete diets during the years that they hunted for food; they could choose what they ate. After domestication, these animals were fed foods that humans ate. With agriculture's development, dogs were fed grain-based diets and developed many deficiencies, as evident in Figure 1.1. Today people know how to formulate and prepare balanced diets using foods for human consumption. It is not necessary to feed a commercial pet food to provide a complete and balanced diet.

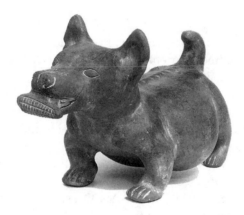

Figure 1.1. Reproduction of ancient Indian figure of a dog living on a diet of corn and showing the consequences of nutritional deficiencies.

What Should a Pet Be Fed?

If a pet food labeled "balanced" or "complete" does not ensure that nutritional needs are satisfied, how should a pet be fed? The answer is not obvious even with the many different commercial pet foods that are balanced and complete. Consider what an animal nutritionist has to say:

> *Because nutritional decisions are multifactorial, often there is no one*
> *simple answer, and there is no one best diet for any species. There is no*
> *one best diet for a dog—the food which is optimal for the puppy is not*

optimal for the adult dog and vice versa. Therefore, to use nutritional science you have to consider all factors involved and weight them accordingly. Thus, there may be more than one solution depending on the weight given to various factors. This makes the application of nutrition frustrating to those individuals who expect "yes-no" answers.[12]

Owners feeding commercial pet foods have no choice but to accept manufacturers' claims. If the balanced and complete claims cannot be trusted, owner-prepared diets should be fed. This gives preparers complete control over diet quality.

Pet Food Quality

Three factors determine pet food quality. Already discussed is a diet's adequacy for required nutrients so that it causes neither deficiencies nor excesses. The source of a food's nutrients is a second factor. What are the food sources for pet foods? Nutritionists agree that producers should use only wholesome ingredients in formulating a commercial pet food. A third factor is nonnutrient ingredients added to improve a product's physical appearance or shelf life.

Manufacturers tell consumers that they can determine a product's quality by reading its label. The U.S. Food and Drug Administration, Federal Trade Commission, and AAFCO establish labeling regulations. These regulations require that labels contain (1) each ingredient listed in descending order of its respective amount by weight and (2) a guaranteed analysis of the minimum amount of crude protein and fat, the maximum amount of moisture and crude fiber, and the added minerals and vitamins. The ingredient list provides *some* useful information for the purchaser selecting a food to feed a small animal pet. However, the label does not give amounts of each ingredient, which, according to regulations, is not necessary. The pet food industry states: "When properly read and understood the pet food label should enable both the veterinarian and the pet owner to make wise judgments on a proper diet for the family pet."[13]

An animal nutritionist's evaluation of this label regulation and usefulness is different.

The required labeling of pet foods, in fact, provides little help to the pet owner. ...

... even for trained nutritionists, the labeling of a product is of limited usefulness in an overall evaluation of its nutritional value. Labels

should produce more information about the digestibility, absorption, and utilization of protein; about the actual amounts of fat and its source, and about carbohydrate, minerals and vitamin content. With this information, the veterinarian can then provide improved service to his clients and protect them from the hazards of attempting to evaluate the information provided by commercial companies or by the label which is currently provided more for sales purposes than for service.[4]

Thus, the guaranteed analysis provides little useful information for making decisions about a commercial pet food. A pet owner cannot know if food described on a label may be a good choice to feed.

■ Pet Food Ingredients

Pet food manufacturers believe that standards of quality are acceptable when the product's ingredients contain nutrient amounts listed on the label. Commercial pet foods contain ingredients that dogs and cats were not designed to eat, however. A representative list of ingredients for dry dog foods shows them to contain, in descending order, ground corn, soybean meal, meat and bone meal, other cereals, and animal fat. Canned dog food ingredient lists show them to contain meat by-products (liver, kidney, lungs, etc.), meat (muscle), cereals (mainly wheat, barley, and oatmeal), and soy flour or grits.

Cereals make up the bulk of dry dog (60 percent) and cat (50 percent) foods. To that primary source of carbohydrate, meat (and bone) meal and soybean products are commonly added as protein sources, together representing up to 30 percent of the diet for dogs and 40 percent for cats. Animal fats, vitamins and minerals, and additives are added to complete the diet. Canned and semimoist foods vary some in the percentages and sources of cereals and protein. It is apparent that dog foods contain nutrients primarily from vegetable sources. Cost dictates the source of the ingredients, but the source is justified by the idea that dogs and cats can adapt to almost any foodstuff making up their diets.

The dog is intrinsically one of the easiest animals to feed, a carnivore turned quasiomnivore through 10,000 years of aping man. This adaptability has permitted the marketing of dog foods that differ widely in ingredients, nutrient composition, and energy density ... nutritional disorders are not likely to be encountered in dogs fed the main types of commercial products in appropriate ways.[14]

Although dogs may have become quasiomnivores, anatomically and physiologically they (also cats) are still carnivores. Their feeding preference is for meat. They have teeth designed to tear flesh and a short and simple gastrointestinal tract, one suited for digestion and absorption of a meat diet. Dogs and cats are not designed for being vegetarians, but they are fed on the premise that they can eat anything humans eat.

Quality is low for most pet food ingredients, however, because their digestibility is lower than food for human consumption. The quality of pet food protein has been studied the most.

■ Quality of Protein in Pet Foods

One commercial company that manufactures drugs for the veterinarian recognizes a lack of quality in most commercial pet foods. Protein is maybe the most important nutrient in pet foods. This drug company criticizes pet foods' protein content by writing the following in its advertising copy:

> However, not all protein sources are of equal value to the carnivore, and the quantity of protein in a commercial pet food often says nothing about its quality. Before domestication, dogs and cats hunted their prey and consumed a diet very high in meat protein, low to moderate in fat, and low in carbohydrates. This diet provided both the proper quantity and quality of protein for the carnivore's unique digestive system. Unlike an omnivore, whose digestive system consists of a fairly large small intestine and relatively small stomach, the carnivore's system consists of a fairly large small intestine and relatively small stomach. Thus, a carnivore's optimum diet must be concentrated, highly digestible, and low in residue because its body is designed to digest primarily protein. If an excess of carbohydrates and fats is included in the diet, much of what the carnivore eats is only partially digested by the time it reaches the large intestine for fecal formation, overloading the digestive and excretory systems. ...
>
> Near the turn of the century, most commercial pet foods included a high percentage of meat protein and were low in carbohydrates, approximating the diet pets ate in the wild. When the Depression struck, however, it became prohibitively expensive to include high-quality protein sources in commercial pet foods. Low-cost, low-protein ingredients were substituted, and fillers high in carbohydrates, such as grains, replaced meat and fish proteins. Thus, pet owners began feeding their carnivorous pets diets better suited to an omnivore's digestive system.

Today, a whole industry has arisen around the production of "better" or "scientifically formulated" pet foods, which attempt to correct the gross nutritional imbalances in generic and off-brand pet foods. However, even the best pet foods, which contain considerable more high-quality protein than generic brands, are not perfectly balanced for maximum nutrition. They may be lacking in certain amino or fatty acids, or contain nutrients in such a low quantity that the animal would have to overeat regularly just to meet NRC minimums. Conversely, they may contain unbalanced excess of other nutrients.

A recent survey compared a well-known canned dog food with the leading dry dog food, both of which claim to provide "balanced" nutrition. The digestibility claim of the canned food was approximately 90%, while the digestibility of the dry food was rated at 80%. The biological value of the protein content (in other words, how useful the protein is to the animal) was given as 69% for the canned food and 60% for the dry. Net utilization (the amount of food used by the animal in relation to the amount provided) can be calculated by multiplying digestibility by biological value. The results: 62% net utilization for the canned dog food and 48% for the dry. This means a dog would have to eat nearly twice the volume of either commercial food to achieve the net utilization that higher, more digestible sources of protein would provide.

Furthermore, a 1984 pet food study revealed that 83% of 78 generic dog foods tested failed to meet NRC standards for analyzed nutrients, and 51% of the samples tested failed to meet their own label-guaranteed analysis. The study further revealed that the growth rate and health of puppies were severely affected when they were fed a diet of nothing but low-priced, dry commercial dog food.[15]

More details of pet food inadequacies are described in the nutrition literature.[11] The pet food industry may believe that the quality of ingredients and the final product are acceptable. However, the last 20 years have shown the pet-owner public that both nutritional and medical disorders developed with the feeding of commercial pet foods.

■ Wholesomeness of Ingredients

The consumer has an additional interest in pet food quality, one that is based on propriety. Pet foods contain ingredients that people will not or cannot eat. Can a quality commercial pet food contain these ingredients and be "wholesome"? Few people are likely to object to a variety of cereals in diets for their cats and dogs. The sources for animal proteins, if known to the consumer, are likely to be objectionable to most, however. For example, meat and bone meal is the second most abundant ingredient for many popular dry pet foods. Most people do not know that meat and bone meal is prepared from (rendered) animal carcasses some days after death. Any animal protein considered inedible for human beings becomes an ingredient for pet foods or for making fertilizer. It is difficult to consider this ingredient wholesome. Commercial pet foods contain unwholesome ingredients.

Summary

What conclusions can be made? The pet food industry tells the consumer:

> *Providing a pet with maximum nutrition doesn't mean merely supplying an adequate daily amount of commercial pet food or supplementing it with treat-type vitamin/mineral tablets. Nor does feeding a pet a scientifically formulated prescription diet ensure that its maximum nutritional needs are met. The fact is that no commercial pet food, no matter how balanced or how high-quality its ingredients, can meet the nutritional needs of every pet. Each animal has its own unique nutritional needs based on age, size, and level of stress. The only way to meet those needs is by supplying a carefully balanced amount of all required nutrients in doses that can be customized for any cat or dog.*[15]

Does this mean that it is difficult to meet an animal's nutritional needs by feeding a commercial pet food?

From the industry's conclusion, one appreciates that nutrition has profound effects on the health and longevity of dogs and cats. So the consumer should have an interest in pet food quality to maintain a pet's normal health. Commercial pet foods can be responsible for health problems. Problems can develop when nutrients are in excess or deficient. That may seem surprising in an era where the pet food industry claims that "more is known about the nutrient requirements of dogs than of man's."[16] Excess or deficiency is more likely for a food's vitamin and mineral or salt content. Major nutrients are also sometimes sufficiently imbalanced to cause health problems. One such problem, hip dysplasia, is more likely to appear in larger breed dogs when their owners enhance growth by feeding foods designed to promote growth. As another example, a commercial canned cat food to manage urinary tract problems contained inadequate amounts of taurine so that some cats developed cardiomyopathy. A variety of these problems are described later.

The quality of pet foods may be the most important factor in many common medical and surgical problems. Gastrointestinal diseases, especially those causing chronic vomiting and diarrhea, represent 35 to 40 percent of all the problems seen in cats and dogs. Before 1950, when pet owners seldom fed their pets commercial pet foods (they fed them mostly owner-prepared foods), the incidence of gastrointestinal problems was much lower than it is now. Skin diseases are common problems in dogs, and their incidence in the past was much lower than it is now. Many skin problems are allergies to something fed; such allergies were infrequent in the past.

Some of these gastrointestinal and dermatologic problems develop because of recommended feeding practices. The pet food industry formulates puppy and kitten foods, but they are nothing more than adult animal formulations containing higher amounts of protein. These commercial foods are usually available to puppies and kittens when their eyes open, about two weeks of age. Common sense if not scientific knowledge tells us to not feed human infants as if they are merely little adults. Instead of feeding diets for adults, parents gradually introduce infants to the large variety of foods eaten by the human adult. The basis for feeding young pets should be no different. Feeding young animals to prevent future medical problems is discussed later.

References

1. Morris, James G. and Quinton R. Rogers. 1994. Assessment of the nutritional adequacy of pet foods through the life cycle. *Journal of Nutrition* 124:2520S–2534S.

2. Grunberg, Rosaly. 1995. Nutrition and disease. *Petfood Industry* 37(5):50.

3. Bryant, Vaughn M. 1995. Eating right is an ancient rite. *The World and I* 10(1):216–221.

4. Newberne, Paul M. 1974. Problems and opportunities in pet animal nutrition. *Cornell Veterinarian* 64(2):159–177.

5. Buffington, Charles A. and LaFlamme D.P. 1996. A survey of veterinarian's knowledge and attitudes about nutrition. *Journal of American Veterinary Medical Association* 208(5):674–675.

6. Garvey, Michael S. 1984. In *Canine Nutrition and Feeding Management*, 2–3. Lehigh Valley, Pa.: ALPO Pet Center.

7. Alpo Advisory Board. 1984. In *Canine Nutrition and Feeding*

Management, 7. Lehigh Valley, Pa.: ALPO Pet Center.

8. Earle, Kay E. and Philip M. Smith. 1993. A balanced diet for dogs and cats. In *The Waltham Book of Companion Animal Nutrition,* edited by I.H. Burger, 45–55. Oxford: Pergamon Press.

9. Simpson, James W. 1992. *Acute Diarrhea in the Dog.* A monograph provided as a service to the veterinary profession by Waltham, world authority on pet care and nutrition.

10. Kronfeld, D.S. and C.A. Banta. 1989. Optimal ranges of actual nutrients. In *Nutrition of the Dog and Cat,* edited by I.H. Burger and J.P.W. Rivers, 27–34. Cambridge: Cambridge University Press.

11. Sheffy, Ben E. 1989. The 1985 revision of the National Research Council nutrient requirements of dogs and its impact on the pet food industry. In *Nutrition of the Dog and Cat,* edited by I.H. Burger and J.P.W. Rivers, 11–26. Cambridge: Cambridge University Press.

12. Morris, James G. 1995. *Nutrition and Nutritional Diseases in Animals,* 1–5. Class Notes for Veterinary Medicine 408, School of Veterinary Medicine, University of California, Davis.

13. Alpo Advisory Board. 1984. In *Canine Nutrition and Feeding Management,* 54. Lehigh Valley, Pa.: ALPO Pet Center.

14. Kronfeld, D.S. 1975. Nature and use of commercial dog foods. In *Diet and Disease in Dogs,* edited by D.S. Kronfeld and D.G. Low, 20–31. Irvine: University of California.

15. *A User's Manual for ProBalance Maximum Nutritional Supplements,* Norden Laboratories.

16. Corbin, J.E. 1972. Nutritional requirements of dogs. In *Canine Nutrition,* edited by D.S. Kronfeld, 1–12. Philadelphia: University of Pennsylvania.

CHAPTER 2
Food Quality and Wholesomeness

Food Selection

Dietary constituents for feeding dogs and cats should be foods with the greatest digestibility and biological value. The digestibility of commercial pet foods is much less than for nutrients humans eat.[1] Efficiency of digestion for human foods is 98 percent for carbohydrates, 95 percent for fats, and 92 percent for proteins. For commercial pet foods these values are no more than 80 percent for carbohydrates, 85 percent for fat, and 80 percent for protein.

A pet's diet can be formulated with basic information on the nutrient composition for all food ingredients. That information provides the content of calories, protein, fat, carbohydrate, fiber, vitamins, and minerals for each food used to make up a diet. The nutrient composition of foods can be found in tables prepared by the U.S. Department of Agriculture or in other sources such as the book *Bowes and Church's Food Values of Portions Commonly Used.*[2] The nutrient content of a certain food often varies, and when precise ration formulation is needed, the tables are not used, and actual analysis of the food ingredient must be done.

Carbohydrates[3-5]

Carbohydrates provide the primary source of energy for most commercial pet foods. The most soluble and digestible carbohydrates are starches and sugars in plants. A starch's source and its degree and type of processing determine its availability. Dogs and cats can almost completely digest and absorb some starch, such as that in rice. More than 20 percent of other starches can escape assimilation. The availability of starch in wheat, beans, and oats is poor. The availabilities of potato and corn starch are also much poorer than that of rice. Of the poorly digested carbohydrate sources, all except potato are the most common ingredients in pet foods. They are the major energy source.

Cooking determines starch digestibility and therefore its availability. Cooking increases the digestibility of all starches, especially raw potato starch, which is poorly digested. Availability of starch to action by digestive enzymes also influences digestibility. Enzymes cannot digest starch inside indigestible plant cell walls. Dietary fiber also reduces carbohydrate digestibility.

With a few exceptions dogs and cats have no established dietary requirement for carbohydrates. After weaning, neither pups nor adult dogs—not even those subjected to hard work—require carbohydrate in the diet. High-carbohydrate diets can reduce fat accumulation in growing puppies.

The natural diet of a true carnivore, such as the cat, is normally very low in carbohydrate, being mainly protein and fat. Blood glucose levels remain normal in carnivores as well as in omnivores but not principally because of the carbohydrates they eat. Carnivores convert amino acids and glycerol for glucose. Cats can maintain blood glucose levels on starvation diets better than other starving animals usually fed high-protein diets. Cats are also able to store more glycogen in their livers than others when fed a high-protein diet.

Dogs usually tolerate dietary starch, and unusual amounts cause few problems, especially after digestive enzyme activities increase and digest greater amounts. Cats tolerate less dietary starch, however, with the maximum not exceeding four grams per kilogram body weight per day. Greater amounts cause diarrhea. Dogs tolerate up to two and one-half times this amount, providing the starch is well cooked.

■ Sugars as a Source of Carbohydrates

Sucrose is sometimes used in commercial pet foods; it is used as a preservative in semimoist foods. Sucrose is found in other foods such as molasses, maple syrup and sugar, honey, fruits, and vegetables. The intestine's mucosal enzyme sucrase hydrolyzes sucrose to glucose and fructose. Cats and dogs have adequate levels of sucrase activity to digest small amounts of sucrose. Excess sucrose is not completely digested and can cause diarrhea.

Lactose is normally found only in milk products but is often used to coat expanded puppy foods. Intestinal mucosal lactase hydrolyzes lactose to glucose and galactose. Lactase activity is usually sufficient to digest small amounts of lactose in diets for adult animals. With little or no lactose in the diet, lactase activity decreases. With subsequent lactose consumption, lactase activity may be insufficient to digest lactose, and diarrhea develops.

Sorbitol is found in fruits and has a sweetening power similar to glucose. Sometimes animals are given foods and medications containing sorbitol. Sorbitol is the alcohol of sucrose. Intestinal absorption is poor for sorbitol, and excessive amounts can result in diarrhea.

■ Carbohydrate Maldigestion[6]

Dogs may not readily digest galactosides, carbohydrates found in dairy products and soybeans. They are digested by intestinal mucosal enzymes unique for galactosides. Enzyme activity may be low if little galactoside has been fed. Feeding large amounts can then cause diarrhea. New foods containing these carbohydrates should be gradually introduced until enzyme activity levels increase.

Longer-chain carbohydrates (oligosaccharides) containing galactose, such as rhamnose, stachyose, and verbascose, form about half the carbohydrate in soybeans. They resist digestion in the small intestine and are fermented by colonic bacteria. Fermentation always produces gas, so flatus is common. Fermentation also produces short-chain fatty acids that support nutrition for the colonic mucosa and promote salt and water absorption. Excess fatty acids can cause diarrhea, however, which is common with feeding excess digestible carbohydrates that the small intestine does not completely digest and absorb. Carbohydrates other than those containing galactose can cause digestive tract upsets when either the amounts in the diet are excessive or there is insufficient enzyme activity for their digestion.

■ Health Problems due to High-Carbohydrate Diets[6]

Feeding high-carbohydrate diets can cause physiological abnormalities and signs of disease. High-carbohydrate diets affect the performance and nutritional state of working dogs. Such dogs cannot maintain normal weight, and their performance as herding, hunting, or sled dogs shows reduced stamina and ability to work.

Diets containing excess carbohydrate that exceeds capacities for digestion and absorption usually cause diarrhea, abdominal distention (from gas accumulation), and flatulence. Poorer digestibility is evident when feeding uncooked carbohydrates and when feeding many of the cereals mentioned earlier. Cooking increases starch solubility and digestibility. Undercooking results in incomplete starch digestion.

Cooking is important to solubilize carbohydrate in soybeans. It is also necessary to inactivate a protein that binds digestive enzymes and reduces protein digestion.

Diets should be formulated with the most highly digestible carbohydrates. Rice is the most completely digested carbohydrate and is economical to feed.

Dietary Fiber[7,8]

Dietary fiber affects carbohydrate digestion and absorption. Dietary fiber consists of plant materials such as cellulose, hemicellulose, lignin, and pectins. Non-plant-cell-wall sources of fiber such as gums, mucilages, algal polysaccharides, and modified cellulose are added to pet foods.

Dietary fibers are insoluble or soluble (Table 2.1). Insoluble fibers consist primarily of cellulose and some hemicelluloses. They also include lignin, which represents a small part of dietary total fiber. Insoluble fibers are the structural building material of cell walls. Insoluble fiber's major source is the bran part of cereal grains. Colonic bacteria do not ferment most insoluble fibers.

Table 2.1. Classification of dietary fiber

Insoluble	Soluble
Cellulose: whole-wheat flour, bran, vegetables	Hemicellulose: psyllium seed
	Pectin: fruits
Hemicellulose: bran, grains	Gums: oats, legumes, guar,
Lignin: wheat, vegetables	barley

Source: Adapted from Bauer and Maskell (1994) and Marlett (1992).

Water-soluble fibers are all other nonstructural and indigestible plant carbohydrates. Soluble fibers such as pectin, guar gum, and carboxymethylcellulose absorb water and form gels; they slow gastric emptying, reduce nutrient absorption, and increase intestinal transit rate.

Increased dietary fiber reduces digestibility of carbohydrates, proteins, and fats and affects absorption for some vitamins and minerals. Water-insoluble fibers such as wheat cereal bran and cellulose reduce digestion and absorption the least.

Fiber increases fecal volume and promotes more frequent defecation. Fiber from cereal grains also increases fecal volume by absorbing water.

■ Fiber Fermentation

Colonic bacteria vary in their ability to ferment fiber. Wheat bran and cellulose fiber are poorly fermented (Table 2.2). Beet pulp, rice bran, and some gums are moderately fermented. Pectin, guar gum, oat bran, and some vegetable fibers are readily fermented. As mentioned, fermentation maintains greater numbers of colonic bacteria and produces short-chain fatty acids, some of which are important for colonic nutrition. Fatty acids also promote colonic salt and water absorption. Excess fermentable fiber results in diarrhea caused by large amounts of short-chain fatty acids.

Fiber added to commercial diets can be completely unfermented, such as cellulose flour, and poorly fermented, such as wheat bran. Neither does little more than increase fecal volume. Some added fibers are jelling agents, such as guar gum and alginates, which are added to canned dog foods that contain gravy and real or simulated meat

Table 2.2. Fermentability of dietary fiber

High	Low	Moderate
cellulose	beet pulp	pectin
methylcellulose	gum arabic	guar gum
wheat bran	rice bran	cabbage fiber
locust bean gum	xanthum gum	

Source: Adapted from Bauer and Maskell (1994) and Marlett (1992).

chunks. Colonic bacteria readily ferment jelling agents, and excessive amounts can cause diarrhea.

■ Fiber Requirements

Fiber has been a component of commercial pet foods during the last 50 years as the trend developed to no longer feed owner-prepared foods. Pet owners rarely add fiber to foods they prepare. Their pets' diets apparently provide adequate fiber to supply colonic nutritional needs. Feeding a mostly meat diet would seem to supply inadequate fiber; however, most of these animals receive adequate fiber because they have few gastrointestinal problems. Dogs and cats in the wild select diets containing negligible fiber. Thus, dogs and cats have low requirements for fiber.

Pet food manufacturers claim that optimal dietary crude fiber levels should range from 1.4 to 5 percent. There is little scientific basis for any recommendation, however. Canine and feline nutrition books devote entire chapters to fiber, but they give no recommendation on dietary fiber levels for normal dogs or cats. An owner-prepared diet contains less than 1.4 percent fiber unless it contains large amounts of vegetables, beans, peas, or bran-rich cereals.

■ Fiber Content of Pet Foods

The type of fiber in commercial diets has been unimportant other than whether it causes diarrhea. High fiber content causing large-volume bulky bowel movements has not concerned most manufacturers. The 20 percent fiber level of some pet foods is excessive. Some manufacturers now add less fiber and use a poorly soluble (so that it does not affect digestive function) and moderately fermentable (so that it provides nutrients for the colonic mucosa but not enough fermentation of fiber to cause diarrhea) fiber. Beet pulp and rice bran are examples of such fibers. If the need for fiber is small, why give an excess that can cause impaired digestive tract function, bulky bowel movements, and diarrhea?

Fiber is the source of energy for colonic mucosal cells. Bacteria accomplish that by producing short-chain fatty acids (acetate, proprionate, and butyrate). More than 70 percent of colonic cells' energy is dependent on these fatty acids. Fiber levels needed to meet these requirements are probably low. Many animals live on very low fiber diets for years without developing colonic disease.

■ **Fiber for Management of Disease**

Fiber is added to commercial pet foods designed for weight reduction. Companies claim this to be effective because fiber reduces digestibility of other nutrients and supposedly reduces appetite or hunger by filling the stomach. Sometimes veterinarians vary the dietary content of fiber for other reasons. They often feed low-fiber diets to dogs with chronic diarrhea. Some recommend feeding high-fiber diets to dogs with colitis, and high-fiber diets can help manage diabetes mellitus in some animals. Although veterinarians promote additional fiber in pet foods to treat these medical problems, there is little scientific evidence that additional fiber is of any value.

Fats[5,9,10]

Animals eat primarily to satisfy their caloric needs. A strictly carnivore's diet contains very little carbohydrate but is rich in fat and protein. Carbohydrates and fats usually provide most of the calories in pet foods; proteins are a minor source of calories. Some dogs are unable to maintain normal weight with low dietary fat.

Fats contribute to a diet's palatability and acceptable texture. They also aid absorption for fat-soluble vitamins. Triglycerides are not essential nutrients for dogs or cats, which have requirements for two or three unsaturated fatty acids, however. Fats are not expensive, but increasing a pet food's fat content increases its cost; therefore, most commercial pet foods are low-fat. Fat in moderation is the most digestible nutrient.

■ **Essential Fatty Acids**

Three essential unsaturated fatty acids required by animals are linoleic acid, linolenic acid, and arachidonic acid. Plants but not animals produce linoleic and linolenic acids. Animals, except cats, produce arachidonic acid by chemical modification of linoleic acid. Deficiency of these three fatty acids results in reduced growth rate, skin problems, and inability to reproduce. Rich sources of unsaturated fatty acids include egg yolks and vegetable oils.

Linoleic acid is the source of omega-6 fatty acids, and linolenic acid is the source of omega-3 fatty acids. Animals need more omega-6 than omega-3 fatty acids for health. However, some scientists believe that the omega-3 fatty acids are important in maintaining health for older individuals. Fish contain higher levels of omega-3 fatty acids (Table 2.3) than most other dietary sources. People who consume large quantities of fish have lower blood cholesterol levels and a lower incidence of heart disease than people consuming foods with lower levels of omega-3 fatty acids.

Even with fish diets animals consume more omega-6 fatty acids than omega-3 fatty acids. Requirements are unknown for these fatty acids and also for any ratio of the omega-6 to omega-3 fatty acids. Some manufacturers suggest the optimal omega-6 to omega-3 ratio to be between 4 and 10 to 1, and a diet with a ratio of greater than 50 to 1 is likely to result in omega-3 fatty acid deficiency. However, no studies prove that omega-3 fatty acid deficiency causes any problems.[11]

The body uses omega-6 fatty acids to make chemicals that promote inflammation. It also uses omega-3 fatty acids to make similar chemicals that may be important in reducing inflammation.

■ Dietary Fat Requirements

Low-fat diets for dogs—less than 5 percent of dry matter total fat and 1 percent essential linoleic acid—leads to dry, scaly skin and harsh coat. High fat content introduced abruptly also may cause problems.

Table 2.3. Omega-3 fatty acid content of omega-3-rich foods

Omega-3 fatty acids (grams) in 100 grams of food[a]					
Salmon	0–1.5	Mackerel	2.2	Herring	1.7
Albacore tuna	0.5	Trout	0.6	Whitefish	1.5
Canola oil	11.1	Soybean oil	6.8	Cod liver oil	19.2
Wheat germ oil	6.9	Butter	1.2	Lard	1.0
Flax oil	57.0[b]				

Source: Adapted from Morris (1995) and Drevon (1992).

[a]Fish contain high amounts of omega-3 fatty acids that require little further chemical modification to form leukotrienes and prostaglandins. Vegetable oils, such as canola, soybean, and flax oils, contain omega-3 fatty acids that require more chemical modification to form the biologically active substances. Moreover, the vegetable oils contain high amounts of omega-6 fatty acids that compete with the chemical reactions changing the omega-3 fatty acids to their active forms. Thus, the omega-3 effects of the fish products are much more effective than those of the vegetables oils.

[b]Flax oil is available at food stores. Capsules containing 1000 milligrams flax oil are inexpensive. Commercial pet foods containing these fatty acids from added fish, and fish oils are expensive.

Undigested fat causes steatorrhea. Excess dietary fat reduces food consumption, which can cause deficiency of other nutrients unless their dietary levels increase. Protein, iodine, and thiamin levels should especially be augmented when dietary fat increases. Excess fat consumption is also likely to cause obesity.

There are no clearly defined optimal ranges for dietary fat levels. A minimum recommendation of 5 percent is usual. The ranges preferred by most dog owners involved with breeding and show dogs or working dogs are considerably higher (15 to 35 percent of dry matter), however.

The normal dog requires linoleic acid at a dietary level of about 1 percent (this is about 2 percent of the calories). Cats have the same requirement. In addition, cats need a source of arachidonic acid. Linoleic acid does not provide that source. Dogs can eat a meat-free diet and receive their nutritional requirements for all unsaturated fatty acids. Cats must eat meat to obtain their arachidonic acid requirements. (There are few exceptions, notably borage oil, red current seed oil, and evening primrose oil, which contain arachidonic acid.)

■ Requirements for a High-Fat Diet

High-fat diets are important for many dogs. Milk fat is the most important source of calories for unweaned animals. Bitch's milk contains about 10 percent fat, which is much greater than cow's milk. Puppies double their body weight rapidly and need calories to sustain that growth and activity. Fat content of queen's milk is greater than cow's milk but much less than that of the dog. With fats providing caloric needs, carbohydrates are less important for energy. Lactose in milk is tolerated well unless for some reason there is insufficient intestinal lactase activity.

High-fat diets are needed to maintain normal body weight in most active larger breed dogs. Many such individuals do not receive enough calories from poorly digested commercial pet foods. They lose weight or are unable to gain weight no matter how much they eat. Dogs working at strenuous activities, such as sled dogs, maintain normal weight by eating high-caloric-density diets.

■ Problems with Feeding a High-Fat Diet

High-fat diets are relatively safe for dogs and cats. Feeding a high-fat diet is thought to cause acute pancreatitis, but that has never been proven.[12] However, many dogs with pancreatitis have a history of eating a fat-rich meal or raiding garbage containing fatty meat scraps. Normal dogs fed a 70 percent fat diet do not develop acute pancreatitis. Some working dogs consume that amount.

High-fat diets cause problems in animals through maldigestion or malabsorption, where unabsorbed fat enters the colon; normally very little fat reaches this point. Bacteria that normally live in the colon transform dietary fats to fatty compounds that are essentially the same as the active ingredient in castor oil (ricinoleic acid). By making one small change in normal fat, bacteria convert it to a potent laxative. Ricinoleic-like compounds damage the colonic mucosa, stimulate colonic water secretion, and stimulate intestinal motility, all of which contribute to diarrhea. Therefore, most diets recommended for the management of chronic diarrhea are low in fat, even for dogs and cats with no loss in their ability to digest and absorb fats.

■ Dietary Fats and Palatability

Dietary fat is important for enhancing palatability. Low-fat diets are unpalatable. The pet food industry works harder to improve palatability than anything else.

For dogs and cats the most important nutritional problem today is not any nutritional deficiency but obesity. Neutering and feeding diets with greater palatability contribute to the problem. Dogs and cats that once ate to satisfy their caloric needs now eat to satisfy their appetite.

Proteins[13,14]

The nutritional value of protein depends on its amino acid composition as well as on the efficiencies of its digestion, absorption, and utilization. The use of amino acids for protein synthesis depends on the availability to cells of all amino acids in the right proportion and at the right time. The diet must provide these amino acids; otherwise, the body mobilizes them from protein in its tissues. Plants can make all the amino acids they require by synthesizing them from simple nitrogenous compounds such as ammonia and nitrates. Animals require most of their dietary nitrogen to be as specific amino acids.

■ Biological Value of Proteins

Biological value describes how efficiently a protein is used. This value is high for proteins from meat, most meat by-products, eggs, and dairy products (Fig. 2.1). Dogs and cats digest these proteins efficiently, and they provide amino acids in proportions suitable for tissue protein synthesis. In contrast, the biological value of most plant proteins is low, due to insufficiencies of specific amino acids and lower digestibility. Careful balancing of proteins from plant sources can improve a diet's protein quality and make them suitable for meeting pets' needs. However, the biological values of pet food proteins are largely unknown. Their value or availability changes when combined with other ingredients and after processing. A nutrient's adequacy and availability can be known only through feeding trials, something the pet food industry wants to avoid.[15]

■ Protein Requirements

The minimum requirement for a protein with an ideal amino acid profile—not generally available on the supermarket shelf—is probably only 5 percent for dogs at maintenance (not working, pregnant, etc.). This estimate is based on a zero nitrogen balance (the animal is neither gaining nor losing nitrogen). Dogs need much more protein, 13 percent for young adults and 19 percent for older dogs, to maintain tissue reserves of protein. Cats need much more protein in their diet. The minimum requirement is 24 percent protein. Most cat foods contain higher levels of protein.

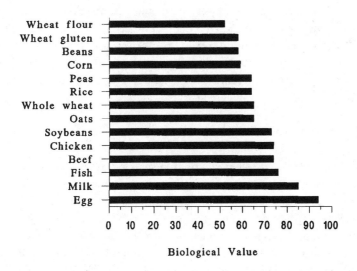

Figure 2.1. Biological values or quality of 14 proteins (adapted from Morris, 1995).

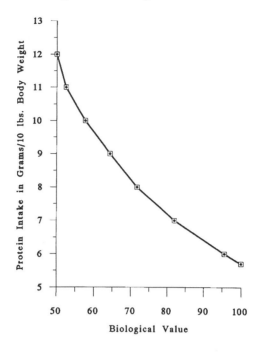

Figure 2.2. Protein needs with proteins of different biological values.

Diets must contain more proteins when their quality (biological value) is lower or when they have less than an ideal amino acid profile (Fig. 2.2). Dog foods contain mixed animal and plant proteins. Because plant proteins are poorer quality, dog foods usually contain proteins at levels of 15 percent for maintenance, 25 percent for growth and breeding, and 30 percent for severe stress.

■ Essential Amino Acids and Nitrogen Intake

Dietary protein is essential for two reasons. It must supply amino acids, which animals cannot synthesize; this makes them essential. Amino acids essential for all animals are leucine, isoleucine, valine, tryptophan, phenylalanine, histidine, methionine, threonine, and lysine. Two additional amino acids essential for cats are arginine and taurine. A complete definition of an essential amino acid is that which the body cannot synthesize at a rate fast enough (from constituents normally in the diet) for normal growth or maintenance. Animals can synthesize seven of the nine essential amino acids (i.e., all except lysine and threonine) from chemical structures normally found in the animal but not in the diet. The body cannot make lysine and threonine; the diet must provide them. Protein is also essential in the diet to supply nitrogen for synthesis of the dispensable amino acids and other products containing nitrogen such as the building blocks of DNA, RNA, and hemoglobin. The body also uses amino acids to make chemicals that serve as regulators of neurologic function and cell growth.

■ Dynamic State of Body Proteins

Adult animals have ongoing requirements for dietary protein because body proteins are in a dynamic state; the body continually degrades and rebuilds them. Some proteins, such as in the gastrointestinal mucosa, turn over rapidly while others, such as in tendons and ligaments, turn over slowly. During protein degradation and rebuilding, the body does not completely reuse the amino acids released. Dietary amino acids replace those lost during degradation.

When caloric intake is inadequate to meet energy requirements, body proteins are catabolized and used for energy. When the diet provides all nutrients needed for energy requirements, amino acids requirements are less, and minimal protein is degraded. During disease with fevers, infection, and trauma, extensive body protein can be lost—much greater than with starvation. Release is augmented for hormones such as cortisone to promote body protein breakdown.

Except during growth the amount of protein or nitrogen in the body should remain stable—the animal is in nitrogen balance. When the intake of nitrogen exceeds excretion, there is positive balance, and the animal stores nitrogen. With a negative balance, body protein is degraded.

Nitrogen balance is not only the result of having the proper amount of protein in the diet. The balance also depends on the quality of protein. To maintain balance, more protein is required when its biological value is low and less when that value is high (Fig. 2.2).

■ Formulation of Diets to Meet Amino Acid Needs

Requirements for dietary protein are based on (1) an animal's nitrogen requirements, (2) an animal's amino acid requirements, and (3) the dietary protein's amino acid composition. Nitrogen requirements are expressed as crude protein requirements. When a diet satisfies these requirements, it is necessary to find the first limiting amino acid. Dietary levels of that amino acid decide the least amount of protein necessary to satisfy all essential amino acids. When a diet satisfies requirements for the first limiting amino acid, it satisfies all other amino acid requirements.

One can evaluate some commonly used cereal proteins for their amino acid content and decide which ones are limiting. Figure 2.3 shows the amino acid content of wheat grain protein and the ratio of the amount contained to the amount required for a growing puppy. The smallest ratio represents the limiting amino acid. Lysine and the sulfur-containing amino acids (methionine is also sulfur containing) are deficient for puppies. A protein containing lysine and the sulfur amino acids, or the amino acids themselves, must be added. To feed wheat without any other protein or amino acids, the amount fed would have to more than double.

Besides calculating the protein and amino acid requirements, it is necessary to determine their availability. The minimal protein requirement is known only after calculating dietary protein's digestibility. Feeding trials give information on protein digestibility; otherwise, it is merely a guess. Moreover, it is not possible to know the efficiency of use for a protein, or its biological value, from amino acid or protein

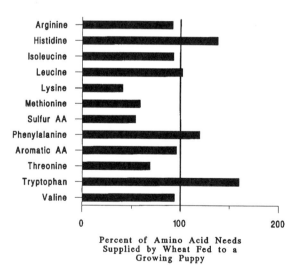

Figure 2.3. Amino acid content of wheat protein showing the limitations due to small amounts of lysine and sulfur amino acids (adapted from Morris, 1995).

analysis of a food. That is determined only by evaluating performance during feeding studies. Digestibility and utilization vary greatly for different proteins. A diet's nonprotein nutrients, such as fiber, influences some of that.

Cooking improves the digestibility of proteins, although sometimes heat can decrease it, especially if protein is cooked with sugars. Heating reduces lysine availability and further reduces its low levels. Processing meat meal and finished commercial pet food products can reduce protein and amino acid availability. The calculated composition can change so the product does not meet an animal's nutritional requirements. Only feeding studies can verify that a diet is complete and balanced.

Wholesomeness

The digestibility and biological value of any pet food depends mostly on its raw ingredients. Government and industry also call for pet food ingredients to be "wholesome." The definition of wholesome is "good for one's health" or "healthful." Wholesomeness has an important effect on digestibility and biological value. Owners preparing pet food can easily select wholesome ingredients to make up their pets' diets. Owners feeding commercial pet foods have little control over wholesomeness of the products.

Because plant proteins are not complete for providing essential amino acid needs, some animal proteins or amino acids must be fed. Animal proteins are more expensive than plant protein sources. The cost of pet foods is lessened by using no more animal protein than is necessary. Using sources of animal proteins not fit for human consumption also reduces the cost. For example, animal meat meals are unfit for human consumption. Some meat meal protein is from animals that died and were beginning to decompose.

Protein sources are the most likely food ingredients to be unwholesome. A pet food is not wholesome when animal products are used that have been produced from dead and rendered animal carcasses. Ingredients listed (and defined by the Association of American Feed Control Officials[16]) on a pet food label that are not likely to be wholesome include meat meal, meat and bone meal, and animal by-product meal.

Meat meal is the rendered product from animal tissues exclusive of any added hair, hoof, horn, hide trimmings, manure, or stomach and rumen contents, except in such amounts as may occur unavoidably in good processing practices.

Meat and bone meal is the rendered product from mammal tissues including bone, exclusive of any added hair, hoof, horn, hide trimmings, manure, or stomach and rumen contents, except in such amounts as may occur unavoidably in good processing practices. It shall not contain added extraneous materials not provided for in this definition.

Animal by-product meal is the rendered product from animal tissues exclusive of any added hair, hoof, horn, hide trimmings, manure, or stomach and rumen contents, except in such amounts as may occur unavoidably in good processing practices.

In contrast protein can be produced from slaughtered animals rather than from carcasses of animals dead for days by using the following AAFCO-defined ingredients:

Meat by-products derived from slaughtered mammals are nonrendered, clean parts, other than meat. It includes lungs, spleen, kidneys, brain, livers, blood, bone, partially defatted fatty tissue, and stomach and intestines freed of their contents. It is suitable for use in animal food.

Poultry by-products must consist of nonrendered clean parts of carcasses of slaughtered poultry such as heads, feet, and viscera free from fecal content and foreign matter except in trace amounts as might occur unavoidably in good factory practice.

Meat is the clean flesh derived from slaughtered mammals and is limited to that part of the striated muscle that is skeletal or that which is found in the tongue, in the diaphragm, in the heart, or in the esophagus with or without accompanying fat, skin, sinew, nerve, and blood vessels.

Poultry by-product meal consists of the ground, rendered, clean parts of the carcass of slaughtered poultry, such as necks, feet, undeveloped eggs, and intestines, exclusive of feathers, except in such amounts as might occur unavoidably in good processing practices.

Slaughtered animals can also provide protein for animal feed when a diseased carcass is condemned for human use. In other cases, protein contaminated with fecal material is condemned but not for animal food. Some protein in pet foods is from animal parts that humans do not consume for esthetic reasons. Some meat sources of protein have nutritional limitations in diets for pets.

Analyses of protein ingredients such as meat and bone meal show great variability. There are virtually no standards, so some products may contain greater amounts of bone than are needed. There is also no analysis on amino acids that meat and bone meal provides when mixed with other foodstuffs. Most nonmeat proteins in pet foods cannot by themselves provide a completely balanced diet. For example, vegetable proteins are deficient in the amino acid lysine. Pet foods need meat products to provide enough lysine. Meat and bone meal is a source of lysine. Heat during rendering to make meat meal destroys lysine, however. Pet food must be analyzed to determine if it contains adequate amounts of lysine. Pet food manufacturers do not say if that is done. Manufacturers can add lysine to meet a pet's nutritional requirements. Larger manufacturers may do that. Smaller ones are not likely to do either the analysis or the addition. Small companies produce a considerable amount of pet food. However, many have a primary interest in making foods for the livestock industry, not in making pet foods.

Foods with predictably high levels of microorganisms or toxins can produce signs of gastrointestinal disease and cannot be considered wholesome. Meat meal is often contaminated with pathogenic bacteria.

Unique Feline Needs[17,18]

Cats have a number of unique nutritional needs, and their diets must be formulated differently from canine diets. Feline diets must provide proteins containing essential amino acids for which cats have an absolute requirement. Dietary proteins must also provide more nitrogen than for most other animals. Cats do not conserve nitrogen as well as other animals. Their enzyme activities for metabolizing amino acids are greater than in other animals, and that activity does not decrease when they eat a low-protein diet. Excess amino acid destruction continues, leaving insufficient amounts for making protein.

Many animals can survive on protein intakes of 4 to 8 percent of the total dietary calories. In contrast, cats need 18 to 20 percent of total calories as protein for growth and 12 to 13 percent for adult maintenance. Thus, cats need two to three times more protein than most other animals under comparable circumstances. The 18 to 20 percent of total calories for a growing kitten represents about 25 percent of the dry weight of the diet. Commercial cat foods contain 30 to 35 percent protein on a dry basis, which is an excess because cats poorly digest the proteins in these diets. Diets formulated for dogs contain too little protein for feeding cats.

Cats cannot synthesize the essential amino acid citrulline, which is low in any food. Cats can convert arginine to citrulline, however, and that means that feline diets must contain arginine to meet the need for citrulline. Cats fed a diet lacking arginine develop hyperammonemia and show clinical signs of illness within several hours. Ammonia accumulates because it is not converted to urea; arginine and citrulline are needed for that conversion. Feline diets must contain arginine.

Cats have only a limited ability to synthesize the essential amino acid taurine from sulfur-containing amino acids. Therefore, a cat's diet must provide taurine. It also helps for the diet to be rich in sulfur-containing amino acids. Diets low in protein, and therefore sulfur amino acids, are more likely to induce taurine deficiency.

Taurine is the most abundant free amino acid in the body. It is not incorporated into body proteins. Its many important functions include being a precursor for bile salts (both cats and dogs have an obligatory and continuous requirement for taurine to make bile salts to replace bile salts lost continuously in the feces). Taurine is also involved in growth and maturation of nervous tissue, maintenance of normal vision, normal heart function, and female reproduction. Taurine is found in all animal tissues but not in plant materials.

Since taurine is free, not incorporated in proteins, in animal tissues, it readily leaches out in water. Cooking meat in water and discarding the water can greatly reduce its taurine content. Proteins from plants such as soybeans and from animal products such as cottage cheese provide no taurine. Canned diets require higher concentrations of taurine to maintain normal levels than do dry foods. No reason is known for this difference other than the two diets have very different formulations.

Within the last decade two diseases, dilated cardiomyopathy and central retinal degeneration, appeared in cats fed commercial diets containing insufficient taurine. (Surprisingly the foods' taurine concentrations were those recommended by the National Research Council.) Only some animals' problems can be reversed with taurine supplementation, so it is important that taurine is adequate in any feline diet. Taurine deficiency does not appear in cats living under natural conditions, catching their own food, or where the animals are eating what nature designs carnivores to eat, meat.

Dry expanded cat foods have a safe taurine concentration if it exceeds 1200 milligrams taurine per kilogram dry matter. In contrast, canned foods need at least 2000 milligrams taurine per kilogram dry matter to maintain adequate plasma concentrations.

Cats show low tolerance for the amino acid glutamic acid. Excess amounts cause sporadic vomiting and thiamin deficiency. Glutamic acid is abundant in vegetable proteins and is comparatively low in animal proteins.

Cats also have some unique vitamin needs. Cats do not have the ability to convert carotene to vitamin A. Lacking the enzyme for that conversion makes it necessary for cats to have vitamin A in their diet. Cats also do not have the capacity for converting tryptophan to niacin. Cats metabolize tryptophan too rapidly to other compounds. The diet must provide niacin. Cats and dogs cannot manufacture vitamin D or its precursor 7-dehydrocholesterol. Thus, the diet must provide vitamin D.

Summary

Dietary carbohydrates are not necessary for most pets. They provide the most calories in commercial pet foods, however. Carbohydrates are the least costly of all nutrients. Carbohydrate-rich foods vary greatly in digestibility, and if they are not properly cooked, digestibility can be poor. The cost rather than the quality of carbohydrate sources dictates which ones are used in commercial pet foods. Low-cost pet foods containing poor quality sources of carbohydrates frequently cause a variety of health problems. Pet owners have little control over carbohydrate quality unless owner-prepared diets are fed.

Fats are necessary for some essential fatty acids. Commercial pet foods fulfill these needs. Fats also can be an important source of calories. Very active larger breed dogs often do not receive enough calories on low- to moderate-fat diets. In these cases it is necessary to feed relatively high-fat diets to maintain normal body weight and the stamina needed for these dogs' physical activity. Obesity is a significant medical problem for a large number of pets. Feeding high-fat diets contributes to the problem. The pet food industry prepares low-fat diets to feed obese pets. The industry prepares some pet foods with high levels of omega-3 fatty acids that are claimed to be effective for treating inflammatory and allergic diseases. No one has shown any benefit from feeding these foods, however. Pet owners completely control the kinds and amounts of fats when feeding owner-prepared diets.

Proteins are the most costly ingredient in any pet's diet.

Commercial pet foods are inexpensive because they are made with cheap sources of protein. The least expensive are grains. Cereal proteins are of the lowest quality, however. Cereals do not provide all the required amino acids, and their digestibility is poor. Pet food manufacturers add meat proteins to provide amino acids deficient in grains. Meat sources used are the cheapest available and often are ones that cannot or will not be used for human consumption. It is important to select wholesome protein sources to feed a pet. That is best achieved by feeding an owner-prepared diet.

References

1. Morris, James G. 1995. *Nutrition and Nutritional Diseases in Animals*, 2-6. Class Notes for Veterinary Medicine 408, School of Veterinary Medicine, University of California, Davis.

2. Pennington, Jean A.T. 1989. *Bowes and Church's Food Values of Portions Commonly Used*. 15th ed. New York: HarperPerennial.

3. Morris, James G. 1995. *Nutrition and Nutritional Diseases in Animals*, 8-1 to 8-9. Class Notes for Veterinary Medicine 408, School of Veterinary Medicine. University of California, Davis.

4. Earle, Kay E. and Philip M. Smith. 1993. A balanced diet for dogs and cats. In *The Waltham Book of Companion Animal Nutrition*, edited by I.H. Burger, 45–55. Oxford: Pergamon Press.

5. Burger, Ivan H. 1993. A basic guide to nutrient requirements. In *The Waltham Book of Companion Animal Nutrition*, edited by I.H. Burger, 5–24. Oxford: Pergamon Press.

6. Williams, David A. 1996. Malabsorption, small intestinal bacterial overgrowth, and protein-losing enteropathy. In *Small Animal Gastroenterology*, edited by W. Grant Guilford, Sharon A. Center, Donald R. Strombeck, David A. Williams, and Denny J. Meyer, 381–410. Philadelphia: W.B. Saunders.

7. Bauer, John E. and Ian E. Maskell. 1994. Dietary fibre: Perspectives in clinical management. In *The Waltham Book of Clinical Nutrition of the Dog and Cat*, edited by J.M. Wills and K.W. Simpson, 87–104. Oxford: Pergamon Press.

8. Marlett, Judith A. 1992. Content and composition of dietary fiber in 117 frequently consumed foods. *Journal of the American Dietetic Association* 92:175–186.

9. Morris, James G. 1995. *Nutrition and Nutritional Diseases in Animals*, 9-1 to 9-9. Class Notes for Veterinary Medicine 408, School of Veterinary Medicine. University of California, Davis.

10. Drevon, Christian A. 1992. Marine oils and their effects. *Nutrition Reviews* 50(4):38–45.

11. Bauer, John E. 1995. Dietary polyunsaturated fatty acids: Progress and prudence. *Journal of the American Veterinary Medical Association* 206(6):768–769.

12. Strombeck, Donald R. and W. Grant Guilford. 1990. *Small Animal Gastroenterology*. 2d ed., 432. Davis: Stonegate Publishing.

13. Morris, James G. 1995. *Nutrition and Nutritional Diseases in Animals*, 7-1 to 7-17. Class Notes for Veterinary Medicine 408, School of Veterinary Medicine. University of California, Davis.

14. Morris, James G. and Quinton R. Rogers. 1994. Assessment of the nutritional adequacy of pet foods through the life cycle. *Journal of Nutrition* 124:2520S–2534S.

15. Sheffy, Ben E. 1989. The 1985 revision of the National Research Council nutrient requirements of dogs and its impact on the pet food industry. In *Nutrition of the Dog and Cat*, edited by I.H. Burger and J.P.W. Rivers, 11–26. Cambridge: Cambridge University Press.

16. AAFCO. 1995. *Official Publication of the Association of American Feed Control Officials Inc.* Atlanta, Georgia.

17. Morris, James G. 1995. *Nutrition and Nutritional Diseases in Animals*, 16-1 to 16-5. Class Notes for Veterinary Medicine 408, School of Veterinary Medicine, University of California, Davis.

18. Baker, D.H. and G.L. Czarnecki-Maulden. 1991. Comparative nutrition of cats and dogs. *Annual Review Nutrition* 11:239–263.

CHAPTER 3
Food Safety and Preparation

Pet Food Contamination

Food is unsafe when it is contaminated with potentially pathogenic microorganisms. Vigilance to prevent feeding such food begins with procurement and is essential throughout preparation and storage. Toxic chemicals also make food unsafe to eat. They can be produced by microorganisms before or after procurement, and many cannot be removed or destroyed by cooking. Some chemicals not considered toxic are used in processed foods to improve appearance, physical qualities, or shelf life. Some animals react to these food additives. Food safety is concerned with preventing illness caused by pathogens, toxins, and additives.

■ Bacterial and Fungal Contamination

Sources
Bacteria and other microorganisms contaminate processed pet foods and can be responsible for digestive tract diseases. The bacteria found consist of microorganisms associated with food ingredients, acquired during handling and processing, surviving any preservation treatment, and contaminating food in storage. Most pet foods are exposed to many potential sources of microorganisms. They include sources of contamination during production, harvest, handling, processing, storage, distribution, or preparation for consumption. Contamination can be by bacteria in soil, water, air, living plants, feed or fertilizer, animals, human beings, sewage, processing equipment,

ingredients, and packaging materials. Contaminated final products can also be a source of contamination for other products.

During the final process of dry food manufacture, the product is coated with a digest of animal proteins and liquid fat (or with lactose for Purina Puppy Food). The digest contains proteins such as chicken viscera. Although cooking destroys any bacteria, the final product loses its sterility during subsequent drying, fat-coating, and packaging stages of the manufacturing process.

Numbers

The number of bacteria in food varies. It depends on original contamination; increases or decreases of bacteria during processing; recontamination of a processed product; and growth or death during storage, retailing, and handling.[1] The usual number of bacteria in most animal products used for food is 1000 to 10,000 per gram. Ground meat is more contaminated than whole cuts of meat because of the type of meat used, extra handling during grinding, and release of meat juices that promote bacterial growth. Bacterial numbers are lower in heated than unheated foods. But poor-quality ingredients, poor sanitation, unsatisfactory heating, recontamination, or poor handling and storage cause some heated products to have high bacterial numbers.

There is great concern today about food wholesomeness. A focus of this concern is contamination of animal-food sources by disease-causing bacteria. People become ill and some die after consuming meat products contaminated with pathogenic *Escherichia coli*. If human foods are widely contaminated, problems of bacterial contamination are likely to be as great for pet foods. The quality of pet food ingredients is poorer than those for human consumption. In addition, animal-protein foods rejected for human consumption are ingredients for either pet foods or fertilizers. Bacterial contamination of rejected food is likely because it is a common reason for rejection. To change this, it would require the industry to completely change the source of important ingredients for making pet foods.

Microorganisms Involved

A study was recently completed to determine the numbers and kinds of bacteria that could be cultured from many commercial dry pet foods. It is surprising that all such foods are contaminated with bacteria.[2] Although only some of those in Table 3.1 consistently cause disease, the widespread contamination of popular brands indicates that feeding a dry food exposes a pet to many different bacteria.

Table 3.1. Bacterial contamination of 40 dog and 40 cat foods

Bacterial Contaminant	Percent of Dog Foods	Percent of Cat Foods
Bacillus cereus[a]	83	78
Other *Bacillus* species[b]	45	52
Enterococcus faecalis[c]	25	15
Ten other bacteria[b]	40	40

Source: James S. Cullor, 1995, unpublished data.
[a]Causes digestive tract disease.
[b]Some can cause digestive tract disease.
[c]Sign of contamination by fecal material.

The numbers of bacteria may not affect most animals that consume a meal quickly. It is predictable that dry foods will cause problems when some of the label feeding instructions are followed. On feeding puppies, one large pet food manufacturer recommends that during weaning, it is best to keep their moistened dog food available at all times. Bacteria in the moistened dry food multiply rapidly, so for puppies that consume the food later, severe vomiting and diarrhea can follow. This is not a recommendation that should be made for a product contaminated with bacteria.

Different species of *Salmonella* are best documented as a bacterial cause of diarrhea in dogs and cats. Salmonella can be cultured from the feces of up to 30 percent of dogs. Many are normal and show no signs of disease.[3] Infection by salmonella usually follows ingestion of contaminated food or water. The food is of animal origin or contaminated by foods of animal origin. Poultry and poultry products are the most frequent source. Other meats and milk are also sources. Salmonella has been found in commercial pet foods, something the public never learns.

It should not be surprising that salmonella has been found in pet foods. A recent notice in the American Veterinary Medical Association journal reported that

> The results of an FDA survey of vegetable and animal protein ingredients used in animal feed, presented at the recent US Animal Health Association meeting, show that nearly 57% of animal protein samples and 36% of the vegetable protein samples tested positive for Salmonella. In other data, more than 60% of animal-protein processing plants and 37% of vegetable-processing plants tested positive for Salmonella.[4]

Pet foods are cooked to kill *Salmonella* bacteria, but where the processing plant is contaminated, food is exposed to contamination after cooking. The chances of contamination with *Salmonella* are so great that some companies routinely culture their final products. If contaminated, the batch of food is not sold for animal consumption. Unfortunately, the assumption is made that commercial pet foods are not significantly contaminated with other bacteria; manufacturers do not culture for others. Other bacteria can contaminate pet foods and be a potential cause for problems, however.

Disease caused by foods contaminated with *Staphylococcus aureus* is the second most commonly identified form of food-borne bacterial disease.[1] The bacteria are most commonly found in contaminated meat, and an important source is food processors. The bacteria produce toxins that cause vomiting and diarrhea. The toxins are exotoxins that directly damage the intestinal mucosa and enterotoxins that stimulate the intestine to secrete large amounts of fluid that cannot be completely reabsorbed.

Staphylococcus aureus contamination can be prevented by using clean food sources. Since food processors are an important source of contamination, adequate hygienic measures should be followed. That might include removing contaminated handlers from the processing operation. Optimum cleaning and sanitizing procedures are necessary. Maintaining food sources under proper refrigeration is essential. Once food is contaminated, the product can be cooked to destroy bacteria, but heating does not destroy toxins that have already been formed so that the food remains a source for gastrointestinal problems.

Clostridium perfringens is the third most common bacterial cause of food-borne illness in humans. This organism is a well-documented cause of gastrointestinal disease in dogs and cats.[5] It is normally found in the intestinal tract of small animals and causes no problems. Under certain conditions it produces spores containing enterotoxin that is released when the spores break open. Food contaminated with *Clostridium perfringens* can be cooked to kill the organism, but its spores usually survive to contaminate commercial pet food. When diagnostic testing is done, enterotoxigenic *Clostridium perfringens* is a common finding in dogs presented with gastrointestinal disease; it can be responsible for chronic diarrhea. Testing is by examining fecal samples for *Clostridium perfringens* spores and by identifying its enterotoxin in feces.

Clostridium perfringens infections are associated with environmental contamination that results in transmission of enterotoxin-producing strains. Many cases develop after boarding at a kennel or during a hospital stay. Whether most of these animals become infected from the premises or from contaminated pet food is unknown. Decontamination is difficult because *Clostridium perfringens* spores are resistant to disinfectants and heat. *Clostridium perfringens* infection requires treatment with antibiotics, and long-term therapy may be required.[5] Dietary management with fiber supplements is reported to be of benefit.

Food-borne infection by *Escherichia coli* is seldom documented in dogs and cats because complicated and expensive testing is required for its identification. *Escherichia coli* is found in the large intestine of normal animals, in a site where the bacteria cause no problems. Some of these organisms are not pathogenic. Others can invade the intestinal mucosa and the body, produce an enterotoxin, or produce an exotoxin that directly destroys the mucosa and causes hemorrhagic diarrhea.[6]

The disease-producing strains may be prevalent, as shown by the outbreaks of *Escherichia coli* infection in people eating inadequately heated meat from fast-food restaurants. Is this a significant problem? In the summer of 1994 a panel of experts met and concluded that "A new, sometimes fatal form of *E. coli* bacteria is now so prevalent in beef that it is no longer possible to guarantee the safety of hamburger. ..." The panel of scientists, policy makers, and meat industry representatives urged some new methods for treating meat before it is sold to the public. It recommended that all ground beef be radiated to kill bacteria. That has not happened yet. Is this applicable to pet foods? All the meats they contain are ground and are probably more contaminated than ground beef prepared for human consumption.

Heating reduces *Escherichia coli*'s ability to cause gastrointestinal upsets by killing the organism and destroying some toxins it produces. The bacteria also produce toxins that are resistant to heat. It is not known whether any commercial pet foods ever contain heat-resistant *Escherichia coli* toxins that survive heat processing.

Escherichia coli in food represents "fecal contamination," and that is more common for some ingredients in pet foods than in foods for human use.[7] For example, meat meal found in many pet foods is prepared from dead animals contaminated with fecal types of bacteria (coliforms). It is possible that *Escherichia coli* is an important cause of infectious gastrointestinal disease in animals. This would make it important to feed pet foods made only from "wholesome" foods.

Other bacteria with the ability to cause gastrointestinal disease include *Bacillus cereus*, *Campylobacter jejuni*, *Streptococcus* species, and a variety of others. Their importance for dogs and cats is unknown.

Fungi are a cause of food-borne illness. They cause disease by invading the intestinal mucosa, allergic reactions, and toxic chemicals produced by fungi. Many toxins are produced by fungi, with aflatoxin produced by *Aspergillus flavus* the most studied. Many foods and feeds contain aflatoxin. Peanuts and corn have been the most significant source. The toxin can cause acute and sometimes fatal problems. The toxin can also cause chronic disease, including cancer, for which the cause is often not recognized. Aflatoxin production in pet food depends on harvest, production, and storage procedures for ingredients and finished products. Prevention is mostly by selection and use of wholesome ingredients and by proper handling and storage to minimize fungal growth.

Food-borne infectious diseases are not commonly thought to be caused by viruses. That may be because little has been done to investigate such problems.

Chemical By-products of Microorganisms

If heat is used to destroy bacteria contaminating food, it is still possible to identify the contamination by chemicals left behind. For example, bacteria acting on the amino acid histidine convert it to histamine, which remains after the bacteria are killed by heat treatment. Measurement of histamine levels in cat foods shows high concentrations in some, reflecting bacterial contamination of ingredients. Other foods rich in histamine include fermented cheeses (very high amounts), pork and beef sausage, some liver, canned tuna, meats, spinach, and poorly stored fish such as mackerel. (Foods can also stimulate the release of histamine in the body. They include egg white, shellfish, chocolate, fish, strawberries, and tomatoes as well as alcohol.)

Many other chemicals formed from bacterial action on nutrients could be used to evaluate food quality. Unfortunately, little is done to assess food quality other than the subjective means of sight, smell, taste, or touch. Measurement of endotoxin levels can evaluate food quality by indirectly determining numbers of endotoxin-producing bacteria in a food before any heat treatment to destroy bacteria.

■ Toxin Contamination

Bacterial Toxins

Bacteria produce many toxins that cause gastrointestinal disease and nonspecific signs of illness. These toxins can be categorized into three types.[6] One attaches to intestinal mucosal surfaces and stimulates secretion of fluid. This enterotoxin can cause massive fluid losses and sometimes death. Heat kills enterotoxin-producing bacteria and usually inactivates their toxin.

Cytotoxins are a second type that can kill mucosal cells directly. Some *Clostridia* bacteria produce this toxin.

Endotoxin is a third type of toxin produced by some bacteria. Endotoxin is formed from part of the cellular structure of gram negative bacteria, such as *Escherichia coli,* normally found in the colon. Endotoxin is released from dead bacteria. Little endotoxin is absorbed in the colon. Endotoxin produced and released in the small intestine can be absorbed and enter the body. Small amounts of endotoxin cause shock that can lead to death.

Endotoxin Effects on the Intestine

Processed pet foods contain endotoxin.[2] Manufacturers do not measure endotoxin levels in pet foods, however, possibly because the amounts are thought to be low. Endotoxin given orally makes normal animals sick.[8] Small amounts of endotoxin cause diarrhea in humans with inflammatory bowel disease.[9] From the few studies that have examined this, endotoxin's mechanism of action is not entirely clear. Endotoxin is known to cause illness by reducing colonic salt and water absorption. It also increases colonic mucosal permeability by releasing mediators of inflammation. Increased intestinal permeability makes it easier for the absorption of endotoxin as well as other substances that can stimulate allergies. Endotoxin acts synergistically with poor protein nutrition to permit the entry of increased numbers of intestinal bacteria into the portal circulation. Thus, endotoxin can initiate and perpetuate damage to the intestinal mucosal surface, and it can perpetuate inflammatory diseases of the digestive system, including allergies.

Endotoxin Effects on the Liver

Endotoxin entering the body is carried to the liver, where it is inactivated. Increased endotoxin levels can damage the liver.[10] Moreover, when the amount of endotoxin reaching the liver is normal, the presence of another potential toxin can interact with endotoxin to damage the liver.[10] The other substances are not necessarily toxins. They include vitamin A, copper and iron, and many drugs. Thus, any level of endotoxin can damage the liver. Exposure to endotoxin should be minimized as much as possible.

Control of Endotoxin Absorption

Antibiotics given orally are helpful in the management of many digestive tract and liver problems in dogs and cats. One beneficial effect of antibiotics is from their activity to reduce numbers of intestinal bacteria and therefore reduce endotoxin production. The potential of endotoxin from the intestine acting with normal levels of substances such as vitamin A or copper to damage the liver is less after giving antibiotics orally.[10] Reduction in endotoxin production also helps protect the lining of the digestive tract. In addition, antibiotics reduce numbers of invading bacteria to which an animal might be allergic.

The diet affects endotoxin production. When nondigestible cellulose or hemicellulose fiber accumulates and ferments in the colon, aerobic bacteria (mostly coliforms) increase 100 to 1000 times.[11] Most pet foods have high concentrations of undigestible matter, thereby supporting aerobic bacterial growth better than other foods. Polished white rice contains low amounts of nondigestible fiber and is more completely digested than other sources of carbohydrate in pet foods. Rice's inclusion in the diet reduces growth of colonic endotoxin-producing bacteria. Thus, it is the carbohydrate of choice in diets for treatment of digestive tract diseases in dogs.

Cultures of lactobacillus are of no value in reducing the numbers of endotoxin-producing bacteria in the digestive system of dogs and cats.

Food as a Source of Endotoxin

In addition to using measures for minimizing the production and absorption of endotoxin in the digestive system, attention should be paid to reducing endotoxin levels in pet foods. In a recent study the level of endotoxin was measured in commercial pet foods.[2] All food examined contained endotoxin. Some contained very large amounts, amounts that were 50 times higher than in foods with smaller levels of endotoxin.

Meat Meal Contaminants

Greater than 50 percent of meat meal can be contaminated with salmonellae.[4] These bacteria produce endotoxin. Processing pet foods containing meat meal by the expansion-extrusion process kills bacteria. Cooking contaminated meat meal does not destroy endotoxin, however, so the final product contains a toxin that can cause disease. Contaminated meat meal is also likely to contaminate other ingredients, including the final product after cooking. Salmonellae sometimes contaminate the premises to the extent that some pet foods containing no *Salmonella*-tainted ingredients are contaminated before the products leave the factory. Recommendations are made to produce animal-protein sources that are *Salmonella*-free and to keep them clean.[4] Other recommendations are to eliminate meat meal materials from feed formulas. However, it is much cheaper to use meat meal than other protein sources. Meat meal is even cheaper than plant proteins.

Meat meal is one dietary source of endotoxin that can make an animal sick. Manufacturers do not analyze pet foods for endotoxin, but it can be present. The fact that coliforms can be cultured from meat meal shows that it contains endotoxin. Meat meals are highly contaminated with bacteria because their source is not necessarily slaughtered animals. Animals that have died because of disease, accidents, or natural causes are a source of meat meal. The animal carcasses may not be rendered or cooked until, sometimes, days after death. During this time, even if the carcass is kept at cool temperatures, bacteria leave the intestinal tract and spread throughout the body. Thus, the carcass is contaminated with bacteria, and high concentrations of endotoxin accompany such contamination.

The pet food industry uses inexpensive sources of protein in order to produce an inexpensive product. Thus, meat-meal protein continues to be used. Some argue that dumping this source of protein is a waste of nitrogenous products that could serve *some* useful purpose. Some suggestions include the use of meat-meal protein to make fertilizers instead of pet food. However, such fertilizers would contaminate soils with disease-causing bacteria. Food for human use could become contaminated by this practice. The solution is to produce animal-proteins that are *Salmonella*-free.

Coliform bacteria such as *Escherichia coli* have been isolated from meat products that cause severe and sometimes fatal diseases in humans. This problem is solved by cooking meat for longer times and maybe at higher temperatures. Because *Escherichia coli* is a coliform, it is another source of endotoxin, however. Heat does not destroy endotoxin, and it can be a cause of illness. So *Escherichia coli* can produce disease by more than one means, with one still potent after thorough cooking. This shows the important need to produce clean meat for both pet and human consumption.

Miscellaneous Food Contaminants

Ingredients for pet foods can contain other disease-causing agents. Aflatoxin is one such that comes from mold or fungi growing on foodstuffs. Mold growth does not occur with proper drying and storage of crops. Pet food plants should control the moisture and humidity of storage areas to prevent mold damage. Proper plant sanitation is also necessary to minimize fungal contamination of pet foods. Heating does not destroy fungal toxins, so they remain in the cooked final product. Ingredients most likely to be contaminated with toxin are peanut meal, cottonseed meal, and fish meal because they originate from areas of the world where there is a high risk for aflatoxin. Pet foods made from such products can be dangerous to feed.

In August 1995 Nature's Recipe, a pet food manufacturer, recalled seven of its dry dog and cat foods made over a two-month period.[12] The products caused many animals to sicken. The company did not state a specific cause but indicated that the products may have contained mycotoxins. The manufacturer blamed the contamination on its source of raw grain. This outbreak shows the importance of using only wholesome ingredients for feeding pets.

Decontamination of Pet Foods

Food is cooked for several reasons. Cooking improves digestibility and kills bacteria that might cause disease. Currently there is great interest in some *Escherichia coli* bacteria that can cause severe digestive tract problems and sometimes death. This occurs because the cooking of meat is inadequate to kill bacteria. The problem is solved by cooking meat longer. However, cooking does not eliminate the problem caused by endotoxin released from the dead bacteria. Endotoxin persists in cooked food when it has been previously contaminated by coliform bacteria.

Drinking water can also be a source of endotoxin released from coliform bacteria that are killed by chlorination. Coliform bacterial numbers reflect the degree of contamination by fecal material in water as well as in food.

Endotoxin contaminates ingredients in pet foods. Meat meal with or without bone is often made from animals that died, animals that were not slaughtered for meat. Coliform bacteria contaminate the carcass used for producing meat meal. Meat meal is processed by cooking to render out the fat and to kill bacteria. Killing large numbers of coliform and other gram negative bacteria releases large amounts of endotoxin. The level of endotoxin in pet foods reflects a food's degree of bacterial contamination before cooking. The level of endotoxin reflects the quality of the foodstuffs that went into the final product. The amount of endotoxin determines whether a pet is at risk for illness when it consumes the food. Nothing can be done to decontaminate a food containing endotoxin.

Pet Food Additives

Pet foods are like all processed foods in that they contain ingredients with no nutritional value. These additives improve a product's appearance or stability. Emulsifiers and surface-active agents keep water and fat from separating. Antioxidants are added to prevent fats from oxidizing, or becoming rancid. Antimicrobial agents reduce spoilage. Added flavors and color improve a product's acceptability by owners and their pets. Some additives are nutrients that the animal absorbs and metabolizes. Examples include sorbitol and ethylene glycol, which retard spoilage. These additives can produce diarrhea, and ethylene glycol can cause anemia in cats.

Most pet food additives are not inert. The small intestine digests and absorbs some of them, and bacteria metabolize many others in the large intestine. The chemical products formed can damage the intestinal mucosa to cause colitis and possibly cancer. The intestine absorbs some of these chemicals, and they can cause disease in other parts of the body.

Some pet foods prepared especially for animals with certain diseases claim to contain no additives. They contain none of the chemicals that must be listed on a pet food label, but they can contain others that do not require documentation on the label, some that can cause problems. For example, dogs can be treated for chronic diarrhea by feeding them a lamb and rice diet. The owner prepares this diet, and when it is effective, the pet has normal bowel movements. The owner may eventually choose to feed a commercially prepared lamb and rice diet. Sometimes this pet food causes the diarrhea to recur, showing that this therapeutic diet contains more than lamb and rice. One or more unstated additives must be responsible for this pet food's failure to achieve the results of the owner-prepared diet.

Most animals remain healthy when fed pet foods containing additives. Consequences of their long-term consumption are unknown. For most healthy pets additive-free foods are not any better, or worse, than foods containing additives. Proponents of the use of additives claim that "... marketing of foods on the basis that they contain no additives or are 'all natural,' is a marketing gimmick only designed to increase sales."[13] On the other hand the use of additives is also a *gimmick* to increase sales (using artificial color and flavors) or to maintain sales (using preservatives) of a product. Preservatives allow a product to sit on a shelf for months before it is fed. One's knowledge of any additives in an owner-prepared diet will always be greater than the information one can find on any commercially prepared pet food. The public learns far more about the composition and safety of an owner-prepared diet's ingredients (almost entirely foods designed for human consumption) than it does about any commercial pet food.

Commercial pet foods contain many additives for improving product appearance and stability (Table 3.2).[14] Additives are not used for nutritional value. Emulsifiers and surface-acting agents are used to prevent separation of fat from water. Added antioxidants prevent fats from becoming rancid, and antimicrobials reduce spoilage. Added flavors and color improve acceptability.

■ Preservatives

Antioxidants—Ethoxyquin

Antioxidants are important additives in processed foods for both human and pet consumption.[15] They are added to retard the oxidation of fats. Animal, fish, and especially plant fats attract oxygen, resulting in their oxidation. This chemical reaction results in rancidity, destruction of vitamins, and production of dangerous chemicals, peroxides. These chemicals can cause disease. Antioxidants effectively and safely slow fat oxidation and peroxide formation.

Naturally occurring antioxidants such as vitamin E and vitamin C (also others such as rosemary leaves) are effective in extending shelf life for many processed foods. Natural antioxidants are more costly and larger amounts are needed compared with chemicals like ethoxyquin. Reduction of fat oxidation consumes naturally occurring antioxidants. Consumption of vitamins to slow rancidity can result in

Table 3.2. Additives in processed foods

Anticaking agents	Flavoring agents, adjuncts	pH control agents
Antimicrobial agents	Flour-treating agents	Processing aids
Antioxidants	Formulation aids	Sequestrants
Colors, coloring adjuncts	Humectants	Solvents, vehicles
Curing agents	Leavening agents	Stabilizers, thickeners
Drying agents	Lubricants	Surface-active agents
Emulsifiers	Nonnutritive sweeteners	Surface-finishing agents
Firming agents	Nutritive sweeteners	Synergists
Flavor enhancers	Oxidizing and reducing agents	Texturizers

Source: AAFCO (1995).

their deficiency. Because vitamin E is unstable (in retarding rancidity; processing of pet foods also degrades it), the more stable form is used, encapsulated acetate ester. Thus, commercial vitamin E added to pet food may not improve stability by reducing oxidation. Ethoxyquin added to pet food spares other antioxidants and by that minimizes vitamin deficiency. Rancidity is less likely in comparison with using naturally occurring antioxidants.

Some question the need for antioxidants in pet foods. A human food such as potato chips fried in fat without any antioxidant is edible for only six days. It is edible 10 times longer when an antioxidant is added. Antioxidants are most important when pet foods contain fats high in unsaturated fatty acids. A pet food with fish oil or vegetable oil as an important source of fat becomes rancid rapidly when no antioxidants are added. Peroxide levels can increase 12 times within 24 hours when such foods contain no antioxidants. Rancidity can reduce a food's metabolizable energy by 15 to 20 percent. Commercial pet foods' processing can significantly accelerate oxidation. Antioxidants are by definition a feed additive, but they are essential for preventing oxidation and preserving a food's nutritional content and quality.

In the 1960s some cat foods were made with fish meal and fish oil without any antioxidants. These diets caused steatitis, a serious and sometimes fatal problem. Adding antioxidants to cat food solved the problem.

Pet foods contain ethoxyquin and a few other commercially prepared antioxidants because they are relatively low-cost and are not consumed as they retard rancidity. Ethoxyquin is safe as well as effective. There is more than three-quarters of a century of study of this chemical. Like almost any chemical if a dog or cat receives enough, it can be toxic. Ethoxyquin has a very wide range of safety, however, and the amount added to pet food causes no problems. Its permitted use as a preservative is 0.015 percent, which is a very low concentration.

Ethoxyquin, more so than any other antioxidant, has anticancer properties. It interferes with cancer induction by other chemicals through actions not dependent on being an antioxidant. Ethoxyquin can bind carcinogenic chemicals and can bind to enzymes that convert inert chemicals into ones causing cancer.

Other Chemical Preservatives
Many other chemical preservatives prolong shelf life for pet foods. Some of these are found in Table 3.3. Ascorbic acid and its salts are preservatives. Butylated hydroxyanisole and butylated hydroxy-

Table 3.3. Chemical preservatives

Ascorbic acid/ascorbate salt	Propyl gallate
Benzoic acid/benzoate salt	Resin guaiac
Butylated hydroxyanisole	Sodium nitrite
Citric acid	Sodium sulfite
Erythorbic acid	Sorbic acid/salt
Ethoxyquin	Sulfur dioxide
Methylparaben/propylparaben	Tertiary butyl hydroquinone
Potassium/sodium bisulfite	Thiodipropionic acid
Propionic acid/propionate salt	Tocopherols

Source: AAFCO (1995).

toluene retard rancidity. (They are the most common antioxidants in processed foods for human consumption.) For most other antioxidants there is little information on any being toxic. An exception is the potential toxic effect of nitrite. Nitrite is used in meat for human consumption, and bacteria can change the chemical to another form with carcinogenic properties, nitrosamines. Very small amounts of this chemical also cause acute and chronic liver damage.

Common preservatives to prevent yeast growth in sugars are sorbic acid and potassium sorbate. Hydrochloric or phosphoric acid is added to make the product slightly acid, which reduces bacterial growth and spoilage. These products generally contain high amounts of coloring matter; red coloring is added to simulate meat and white (titanium dioxide) to simulate fat. The final product looks like meat and fat.

■ Additional Special-Purpose Products

Many substances are available for the purposes listed in Table 3.2. Examples are in Table 3.4. Most of the materials or chemicals are inert and cause no problems. Others can be toxic at levels much higher than usually found in processed foods. It is apparent that most of the substances control the physical characteristics (i.e., the appearance) of pet foods. Thus, these substances are rarely found in diets prepared by a pet owner.

The list in Table 3.4 is only partial. Many other materials are found in pet foods, and some can cause problems. An example of such an

Table 3.4. Special-purpose ingredients

Ingredient	Purpose
Aluminum sulfate	Antigelling agent
Attapulgite clay	Anticaking agent
Ball clay	Pelleting agent
Calcium stearate	Anticaking agent
Diatomaceous earth	Inert carrier
Disodium EDTA	Solubilizer
Ethoxylated fats	Emulsifier
Ethyl cellulose	Binder or filler
Guar gum	Stabilizer
Iron ammonium citrate	Anticaking agent
Kaolin	Anticaking agent
Locust bean gum	Stabilizer
Mineral oil	Lubricant
Monosodium glutamate	Seasoning
Phosphoric acid	Miscellaneous
Polysorbate	Emulsifier
Propylene glycol	Emulsifier
Pyrophilite	Carrier
Saccharin sodium	Sweetener
Talc	Lubricant
Tetra sodium phosphate	Dispersant
Titanium oxide	Color additive
Xanthum gum	Thickener
Yellow prussite of soda	Anticaking agent

Source: AAFCO (1995).

ingredient, carrageenan, made from seaweed, is a carbohydrate that can cause intestinal inflammation. Some pet foods contain carrageenan to produce a desired physical quality. Some pets react to commercial pet foods with persistent digestive tract disturbances. It is possible that carrageenan in some pet foods is responsible for inducing inflammation resulting in digestive tract disease.

Unique Feline Food and Additive Intolerances

Cats are more sensitive to food additives than other animals. Cats are intolerant to the common food preservative benzoic acid. Benzoic acid occurs naturally in plants but is not found in animal tissues. Cats have a limited ability to metabolize the chemical to a form that their bodies can excrete. Aspirin is a form of benzoic acid that cats excrete poorly.

Cat foods can contain propylene glycol, which can damage erythrocytes. The result is a shorter life span that can lead to anemia. Propylene glycol shortens life span for erythrocytes, which can lead to anemia.

Relatively small amounts of onions can poison cats. Documented cases appeared after cats ate onion soup and baby foods containing onion as a flavoring agent.

Cocoa and chocolate can poison dogs, and the toxic derivative, theobromine, can be lethal for cats.

Cats may have other unique intolerances that are currently unknown. Feline hyperthyroidism has been associated with feeding commercial canned cat food. This disease may be related to some food additives or to cats' unique needs that are not being met.

Pet Food Preparation

Food selection is the essential first step in practicing food safety. Food handling and preparation procedures determine whether or not the final diet is safe for consumption. Owners control food safety when they prepare diets themselves. They have no control over the safety of any commercially prepared or processed foods.

The U.S. Department of Agriculture Food Safety and Inspection Service (FSIS) has established a farm-to-table approach to improve the safety of meat and poultry at each step in the food production, distribution, and marketing chain. After the consumer purchases these foods, the FSIS gives a number of reasons for handling food safely.[16] Most importantly, safe food handling prevents illness and can save a pet's life. Owners preparing a pet's diet have a responsibility to the animal to handle food safely, and this also saves money. Safe food handling is easy, and its practices are the ones most likely to preserve food's peak quality. Growth of microorganisms is reduced, and quality of food appearance, flavor, and texture is maintained. Nutritional benefits are not lost, and food need not be discarded because of decay or temperature abuse.

Safe handling of food by consumers begins in the store and continues in the home. The important practices of handling include purchasing, storing, prepreparation, cooking, serving, and handling leftovers. Safe handling prevents or minimizes hazards associated with biological (bacteria), chemical (cleaning agents), and physical (equipment) causes.

Meat and poultry products should be purchased last during shopping, and packages of raw meat and poultry should be kept separate from other foods, especially ones eaten without further cooking. Plastic bags should be used to enclose individual packages of meat.

Home storage of meat should be in a refrigerator at temperatures below 40°F or in a freezer at a temperature of 0°F. Most food-borne bacteria grow slowly at 40°F and do not grow at 0°F. Meat should be refrigerated or frozen immediately at home. Juices from raw meat must not be permitted to drip on other refrigerated foods. Hands should be washed with soap and water for 20 seconds before and after handling any raw meat, poultry, or seafood product. According to the Centers for Disease Control (CDC), hand washing is the single most important means of preventing the spread of infection from bacteria, pathogens, and viruses causing disease and food-borne illness. Canned foods should be stored in a cool, clean, dry place, not subject to extreme cold or heat. Foods should not be stored under a sink or directly on the floor; they should be stored separate from any cleaning supplies.

Prepreparation most importantly includes hand washing done before and after food handling. It is essential after prepreparation is interrupted by the handler touching animals or blowing his or her nose. Juices from raw meats should not contaminate other foods that will not be cooked before eaten. In addition to hand washing, counters, equipment, utensils, and cutting boards should be sanitized with a chlorine solution of one teaspoon liquid household bleach per quart of water. Frozen foods should never be thawed at room temperature; thawing is done in the refrigerator. Foods can be thawed in the microwave if they are cooked immediately. Thawing can also be done in cold water in an airtight plastic wrapper or bag, with the water changed every 30 minutes until the food is thawed.

Food must always be cooked thoroughly, which destroys any pathogenic bacteria. Freezing or rinsing food in cold water is unacceptable for destroying bacteria. Beef products should be cooked to at least 160°F to destroy *Escherichia coli* and other pathogenic bacteria. Poultry and pork products should be heated to at least 170°F to destroy *Salmonella* and other pathogens. It may be safest to heat to 180°F. (As an example, bringing to a boil and simmering chicken thighs for one hour is more than enough to kill all bacteria.) A meat thermometer can be used to verify that this temperature is reached. Meat products should be cooked thoroughly the first time, and then they may be refrigerated and safely reheated later. Never cook them partially and then complete cooking later. Never refrigerate partially cooked products. Microwaving foods should be done following the manufacturer's instructions and using microwave-safe containers and procedures to ensure thorough cooking.

Food is handled for serving only after hands are washed with soap and water. Food should be served in clean dishes or containers. Foods should not be allowed to stand for appreciable lengths of time between 40°F and 140°F, a temperature zone in which bacteria multiply rapidly. This time should not exceed two hours at room temperature and a maximum of one hour on hot days at 90°F.

Leftovers can be handled before and after hand washing. Clean utensils and dishes should be used. Leftovers should be divided into small units and stored in shallow containers for quick cooling. They should be refrigerated within two hours of cooking. Foods left out too long should be discarded. Leftovers should be reheated thoroughly to a temperature of 165°F or until hot and steamy. If there is any question about the safety of leftovers, they should be discarded.

Summary

Government and industry call for pet food ingredients to be wholesome. The definition of wholesome is "good for one's health" or "healthful." Foods with predictably high levels of microorganisms or toxins can produce signs of gastrointestinal disease and cannot be considered wholesome. They should not be used to produce food for pets.

Bacteria live in the small intestine, and they represent the retention of orally ingested bacteria.[17] The kinds and numbers of bacteria living there change as the population of ingested bacteria change. Bacteria are contaminants of food and/or environment. The contamination of the small intestine can be controlled by using wholesome foods and proper processing for producing pet foods. Recent studies show that the bacterial population of the small intestine can be reduced slightly by the addition of some novel, complex, nondigestible carbohydrates to pet food.[18] Use of such substances to prevent the consequences of bacterial contamination of pet foods should not replace efforts to produce a product with wholesome ingredients.

In summary, commercial pet foods contain many additives. Some must be listed on the label. Many others need not be listed. Food additives can cause health problems. Very few are proven to cause problems, however. For many of the others it is difficult to prove any harmful effects. No doubt, some of these chemicals can interact with others to synergistically damage cells in different parts of the body.

Medical problems sometimes disappear when pets are fed owner-prepared diets but return when the same ingredients used in these diets are fed in the form of a specially prepared commercial pet food. In such cases a pet food additive may be responsible for the health problem.

References

1. Banwart, George J. 1989. *Basic Food Microbiology.* New York: Van Nostrand Reinhold.

2. Cullor, James S. 1995. Unpublished data.

3. Borland, Edith D. 1979. Salmonella infection in dogs, cats, tortoises and terrapins. *Veterinary Record* 96(18):401–402.

4. Anonymous. 1995. Food notes on immunosuppression: *Salmonella. Journal of the American Veterinary Medicine Association* 206:935.

5. Twedt, David C. 1993. Canine *Clostridium perfringens* diarrhea. In *Proceedings of 17th Waltham/OSU Symposium on Gastroenterology,* 28–32. Vernon, Calif.: Waltham.

6. Strombeck, Donald R. and Grant Guilford. 1990. *Small Animal Gastroenterology.* 2d ed., 320–327. Davis: Stonegate Publishing.

7. Hollingsworth, Jill and Bruce Kaplan. 1997. Zero tolerance for visible feces helps FSIS fight foodborne pathogens. *Journal of the American Veterinary Medicine Association* 211(5):534–535.

8. Cort, N., G. Fredriksson, H. Kindahl, L.-E. Edqvist, and R. Rylander. 1990. A clinical and endocrine study on the effect of orally administered bacterial endotoxin in adult pigs and goats. *Journal of Veterinary Medicine* 37: 130–137.

9. Ciancio, Mae J. 1994. Endotoxin-induced diarrhea in inflammatory bowel disease: Cellular and molecular mechanisms. *Progress Inflammatory Bowel Disease* 15(1):17.

10. Strombeck, Donald R. and Grant Guilford. 1990. *Small Animal Gastroenterology,* 2d ed., 519–521. Davis: Stonegate Publishing.

11. Strombeck, Donald R. and Grant Guilford. 1990. *Small Animal Gastroenterology,* 2d ed., 18–19. Davis: Stonegate Publishing.

12. Anonymous. 1995. Nature's Recipe recall lost $20 million due to vomi-

toxin. *Petfood Industry* 37(6):37–38.

13. Lewis, Lon D., Mark L. Morris, Jr., and Michael S. Hand. 1987. *Small Animal Clinical Nutrition III.* 3d ed. Topeka: Mark Morris Associates.

14. AAFCO. 1995. *Official Publication of the Association of American Feed Control Officials Inc.* Atlanta, Georgia.

15. Hilton, J.W. 1989. Antioxidants: Function, types and necessity of inclusion in pet foods. *Canadian Veterinary Journal* 30:682–684.

16. Anonymous. 1997. Food Safety and Inspection Service. U.S. Department of Agriculture, Washington, D.C. (Internet).

17. Willard, M.D., R.B. Simpson, T.W. Fossum, N.D. Cohen, E.K. Delles, D.L. Kolp, D.P. Carey, and G.A. Reinhart. 1994. Characterization of naturally developing small intestinal bacterial overgrowth in 16 German shepherd dogs. *Journal of the American Veterinary Medicine Association* 204:1201–1206.

18. Willard, M.D., R.B. Simpson, K. Delles, N.D. Cohen, T.W. Fossum, E.D.L. Kolp, and G.A. Reinhart. 1994. Effects of dietary supplementation of fructo-oligosaccharides on small intestinal bacterial overgrowth in dogs. *American Journal of Veterinary Research* 55:654–659.

PART TWO

Feeding Normal Dogs and Cats

CHAPTER 4
Canine and Feline Energy Requirements

Energy Requirements

■ Basal Metabolic Requirements

All animals require a source of energy, something essential to life. They need energy to support indispensable work in cells and organs. The energy required for this work represents resting or basal metabolic rate. Besides this energy expenditure, animals need a source of energy for muscular activity, stress, heat production to maintain body temperature, and all the processing of a meal. This additional energy requirement is sometimes called thermogenesis. The resting metabolic rate accounts for a little more than one-half of the total, with most of that used by functions in the liver. It may seem that muscle activity should account for a major part of the total energy requirement. Skeletal muscle that accounts for about one-half of the body's mass is dependent on only 20 percent of the energy needs under normal conditions, however.

An animal's basal metabolic rate does not normally change. So it does not impact energy requirements. Thermogenesis often changes and is responsible for changes in energy requirements. When the energy intake does not change to match an animal's requirements, there is a gain or loss of weight.

An animal's energy needs are based on its body weight. The calculation of this requirement is also based on the body surface area because that more accurately accounts for heat loss. (Surface area may correlate better because it is a more accurate reflection of the size of the metabolically active tissues of the body.) The energy requirement per pound of body weight is greatest for very small breed animals and least for the large.

■ Food's Available Energy—Food Digestibility

No animal can use all the energy in its food. The percent used depends on the animal's completeness of digestion, absorption, and use for any food. Digestible energy is the percent of a food's total energy available after digestion and absorption. An animal does not use all of its digestible energy; what it uses is metabolizable energy. It is most useful to describe a diet's energy value in terms of metabolizable energy. Animals regulate their food intake by eating to satisfy metabolizable energy requirements. Pet foods vary greatly in the usable energy they provide any individual animal.

■ Daily Caloric Requirements—Determinants

An adult dog's energy requirements can be calculated by finding its normal body weight and using Table 4.1. The daily needs are for a moderately active dog living in a temperate climate. The table's values are 94 to 95 percent of the National Research Council (NRC) recommendations. Some studies show the NRC recommendations overestimate the caloric needs of the average canine house pet.[1] The average daily caloric needs of different groups of dogs range from a low of 78 percent to a high of 94 percent of the NRC recommendation. Other studies report that the recommended values in the literature overestimate the energy requirement for maintenance of dogs, with the overestimations ranging from 10 to 60 percent. The recommendations in Table 4.1 may provide more calories than some pets need to maintain normal weight.

An animal's age influences its caloric needs.[1] Adult dogs below two years of age need 10 to 20 percent more calories than dogs between three and seven years. Dogs older than seven years need about 20 percent less energy than dogs between three and seven years of age. Less food should be fed as an animal ages.

Caloric requirements also show some breed differences.[2] Based on requirements per pound of body weight, the Newfoundland has lower energy requirements than six other breeds of different sizes from

Table 4.1. Daily caloric requirements for adult dogs

lb	kcal	lb	kcal	lb	kcal	lb	kcal	lb	kcal	lb	kcal
1	70	31	908	61	1508	91	2035	121	2520	151	2976
2	115	32	929	62	1526	92	2052	122	2536	152	2990
3	157	33	951	63	1545	93	2069	123	2551	153	3005
4	195	34	973	64	1563	94	2085	124	2567	154	3020
5	231	35	994	65	1581	95	2102	125	2582	155	3034
6	265	36	1015	66	1599	96	2119	126	2598	156	3049
7	297	37	1036	67	1618	97	2135	127	2613	157	3064
8	329	38	1057	68	1636	98	2151	128	2629	158	3078
9	359	39	1078	69	1654	99	2168	129	2644	159	3093
10	389	40	1099	70	1672	100	2184	130	2660	160	3108
11	417	41	1119	71	1690	101	2201	131	2675	161	3122
12	445	42	1140	72	1707	102	2217	132	2690	162	3137
13	473	43	1160	73	1725	103	2233	133	2705	163	3151
14	500	44	1180	74	1743	104	2249	134	2721	164	3166
15	526	45	1200	75	1760	105	2266	135	2736	165	3180
16	553	46	1220	76	1778	106	2283	136	2751	166	3195
17	578	47	1240	77	1796	107	2298	137	2766	167	3209
18	604	48	1260	78	1813	108	2314	138	2781	168	3223
19	629	49	1279	79	1831	109	2330	139	2796	169	3238
20	653	50	1299	80	1848	110	2346	140	2811	170	3252
21	677	51	1318	81	1865	111	2362	141	2826	171	3267
22	702	52	1338	82	1882	112	2378	142	2842	172	3281
23	725	53	1357	83	1899	113	2394	143	2857	173	3295
24	749	54	1376	84	1916	114	2410	144	2872	174	3309
25	772	55	1395	85	1934	115	2426	145	2887	175	3324
26	795	56	1414	86	1951	116	2442	146	2902	176	3338
27	818	57	1433	87	1968	117	2457	147	2916	177	3352
28	841	58	1452	88	1985	118	2473	148	2931	178	3366
29	863	59	1471	89	2002	119	2489	149	2946	179	3381
30	886	60	1489	90	2019	120	2504	150	2961	180	3395

Source: Data are calculated from Burger (1993).

Note: For each pound greater than 180 pounds, add 4 kilocalories per pound of additional weight. The values in this table are for dogs living in a temperate climate and with a moderate amount of physical activity. Calculations were made with this formula: kilocalories/day = $125 \times$ body weight$^{0.75}$.

dachshunds to Great Danes. The Newfoundland's requirements are about 17 percent less.

It is obvious that animals performing strenuous work or engaged in considerable physical activity require more energy. Some very active dogs cannot maintain their normal weight when fed standard commercial pet foods. They require additional energy, and that is most often provided by feeding a high-fat diet. The energy requirements for some of these dogs can be tremendous, with the working energy needs for sled dogs, for example, increasing eight times over their resting needs.[3]

Determination of an Adult Dog's Caloric Needs

The daily caloric requirements for an individual animal depend on its physiological state, such as adult maintenance, growth, pregnancy, or lactation. Other determining factors include the animal's activity and temperament, environmental temperature, and the diet's digestibility. Calculations of the caloric needs are based on an adult animal's body weight as follows.

Maintenance needs for a dog based on NRC recommendations:

$$\text{Body weight}^{0.75} \times 132 = \text{Kilocalories needed} \tag{4.1}$$

Note that this calculation will result in a 5 to 6 percent higher amount of calories than found in Table 4.1.

Maintenance needs for a dog based on Waltham Centre for Pet Nutrition (WCPN) recommendations:

$$\text{Body weight}^{0.75} \times 125 = \text{Kilocalories needed} \tag{4.2}$$

The WCPN formula[4] is used to compile the caloric requirements found in Table 4.1. The figures calculated are for the average, moderately active adult dog that lives in a thermoneutral environment. Less active dogs require considerably fewer calories per day. Extremes in temperature, illness, or physical activity, such as racing or hunting, can increase the daily caloric needs by 300 percent or more.

Calculation of energy requirements provides figures that are the most precise measures for the "average" dog in different physiological states. Since many dogs differ from the average, these formulas serve as a guide for establishing a starting point for any feeding program. On any feeding program animals should be weighed at frequent intervals (weekly) to evaluate appropriateness of measurements and for adjusting caloric intake.

■ **Feeding Commercial Dog Food to Meet Caloric Requirements**

Pet food labels do not report the number of calories a food provides per unit or pound (in contrast to most foods for human consumption that list caloric content). Caloric content can be learned from the company (companies print toll-free 800 numbers on pet food packages).

Most pet owners feeding commercial pet foods have no knowledge how many calories are fed. It is difficult to calculate the appropriate number of calories, even by using the formulas and tables in this chapter. Commercial pet food labels give feeding instructions that make it even more difficult to know how much to feed adult dogs. Feeding instructions found on any pet food label describe a broad range of cups of food to feed a dog depending on its size. The range of cups is usually so great that one has to guess at whether a pet eats the correct amount of food to meet its requirements. Following is a pet food manufacturer's conclusion on feeding advice.

> *Most manufacturers of pet food include feeding instructions on the package label. Some labels recommend daily intakes that are about 20 percent higher for smaller dogs and up to 70 percent higher for larger dogs than the average values given in Table 2. This is usually done to ensure that all dogs will receive their needs but it may lead to overfeeding for most dogs. Overfeeding for whatever reason is conducive to obesity in older dogs and perhaps skeletal problems in young, growing dogs.[5]*

The most effective way to determine how much to feed is to first calculate an animal's energy requirements from Table 4.1. Then feed an amount of food to supply its caloric needs. Because commercial pet food labels do not state caloric content, it is necessary to phone the company or calculate the caloric content as described above. For the recipes in this book, the caloric content is given. Most recipes also state what size dog or cat a given amount will sustain.

Determination of a Growing Dog's Caloric Needs

The NRC arbitrarily established the following formulas to determine caloric needs for growing dogs.

Needs for puppies from weaning to 50 percent of adult weight:

Body weight$^{0.75}$ × 264 = Kilocalories needed   (4.3)

Needs for puppies from 51 percent of adult weight to adult weight:

Body weight$^{0.75}$ × 198 = Kilocalories needed   (4.4)

These formulas imply that caloric needs are relatively constant during the initial part of the growth, up to 50 percent of adult weight. Then a different, lesser need suffices for the remainder of growth. However, the figure 264 in formula 4.3 is not constant. For the first half of this growth phase, the requirement is well over 300 per kilogram body weight$^{0.75}$. For many breeds it remains over 300 well into the last phase of growth. Furthermore, the value changes throughout each period; it is not constant at any time. These formulas will lead to underfeeding during the beginning of each growth period and overfeeding during the end of each growth period.

For puppies that will mature to become large or giant breed dogs, some experts recommend caloric amounts that are 15 to 17 percent less than their NRC established requirements. This creates controversy because some nutritionists believe that puppies fed no more energy than NRC recommendations are too lean. Some nutritionists, at an international symposium on nutrition for dogs and cats, summarized this difference of opinion as follows:

> *Growing puppies of a given breed require about two to three times as much energy per unit bodyweight as adult dogs of the same breed. The US National Research Council suggests feeding twice as much energy per unit bodyweight of an adult dog to the newly weaned puppy (NRC 1985). A purely arbitrary decrease to 1.6 times maintenance is recommended when 40 percent of adult bodyweight is achieved and 1.2 times maintenance when 80 percent of adult weight is reached. This reduction will compensate for the decline in energy requirement from weaning to maturity. Our experience indicates that feeding strictly in accordance with the NRC energy scale produces puppies which tend to be rather lean, compared with what is generally accepted by dog breeders.*[6]

What is necessary to feed growing dogs to produce individuals that the dog breeders prefer?

Pet food manufacturers recommend feeding growing dogs more than the NRC recommends. Feeding those amounts produces the kind of animals breeders and owners prefer. They follow the pet food manufacturers' recommendation that "the dog owner should feed the animal so that its size, condition and general appearance are pleasing to his eye."[5] Unfortunately, if this recommendation is followed, puppies will suffer from overnutrition and the possibility of orthopedic problems.

Obviously a pet food producer does not want to recommend feeding puppies at a level that will make them appear lean and unthrifty. Consequently they recommend greater food intakes compared with those recommended by the NRC. In studies on growing dogs, pet food manufacturers feed up to 30 percent more energy than that recommended by the NRC. A company's feeding instructions will be based on results from these studies.

There is no question that determining the caloric needs of growing dogs is more difficult than deciding how much to feed adult dogs. Growing dogs are of different sizes, and their needs change as they mature, so feeding them is often no more than a guess. If one follows the recommendation to reduce a puppy's energy intake by 15 percent below NRC recommendations, the amount fed will be much less than a pet food label suggests feeding. Table 4.2 gives the caloric needs of different size growing dogs at any given age and weight. If the caloric content of commercial pet food is known, a good estimation can be made on how much to feed. It is virtually impossible to estimate a puppy's caloric needs from information on pet food labels, however. These labels give no information on caloric content per ounce or per cup of food.

Pet food labels recommend amounts to feed in a range of cups to give at a certain age and for a puppy that will mature to a given weight range. The range of cups to feed varies greatly so that a two- or three-month-old puppy estimated to weigh over 100 pounds at maturity should eat from three to six cups of a dry puppy food. Also, if puppies gain one-third or one-half of their adult weight at three months for one breed and at six months for another breed, their food requirements per pound of body weight will be greatly different. Dogs that are still growing after one year of age will need more than those of comparable weight that stopped growing at eight months of age. This is confusing and shows that calculating how much food to feed a puppy is no more than a guess. One result is for pet owners to feed puppies free-choice; the puppy decides how much food is needed. The result is puppies overeating and suffering from overnutrition. Some nutritionists agree that determining how much to feed is no more than a guess: "No exact amount of food can be prescribed. Instead, warning should be given against overfeeding, or any abrupt change in the diet."[7]

No matter how the needs of a puppy is determined, it is most

Table 4.2. Daily caloric requirements for growing dogs with estimated adult body weight of 10–175 pounds

	Estimated Adult Body Weight					
	10 Pounds		20 Pounds		30 Pounds	
Age (Months)	Weight (Pounds)	Caloric needs	Weight (Pounds)	Calorie needs	Weight (Pounds)	Caloric needs
2	4.0	306	6.0	500	8.3	668
3	5.6	324	8.0	522	12.5	705
4	6.6	342	11.0	550	15.6	747
6	7.8	351	13.7	589	19.8	792
9	8.9	374	16.3	628	23.0	828
12	10.0	389	18.8	637	26.7	855
Adult	10.0	389	20.0	653	30.0	886

	Estimated Adult Body Weight					
	40 Pounds		50 Pounds		60 Pounds	
Age (Months)	Weight (Pounds)	Caloric needs	Weight (Pounds)	Calorie needs	Weight (Pounds)	Caloric needs
2	10.0	792	12.0	935	14.0	1080
3	15.6	851	19.0	1025	23.0	1224
4	19.6	923	24.0	1116	29.0	1368
6	25.2	968	30.0	1118	36.0	1295
9	29.4	979	36.0	1134	43.0	1331
12	34.0	1106	41.0	1260	50.0	1475
Adult	40.0	1099	50.0	1299	60.0	1489

	Estimated Adult Body Weight					
	70 Pounds		80 Pounds		90 Pounds	
Age (Months)	Weight (Pounds)	Caloric needs	Weight (Pounds)	Calorie needs	Weight (Pounds)	Caloric needs
2	15.0	1188	18.0	1350	18.0	1350
3	26.0	1434	30.0	1639	32.0	1761
4	33.0	1597	38.0	1825	41.0	1943
6	42.0	1458	48.0	1666	52.0	1802
9	49.0	1457	56.0	1665	63.0	1844
12	57.0	1647	65.0	1883	73.0	2064
Adult	70.0	1672	80.0	1848	90.0	2019

Table 4.2. *(cont.)*

	Estimated Adult Body Weight					
	100 Pounds		110 Pounds		120 Pounds	
Age (Months)	Weight (Pounds)	Caloric needs	Weight (Pounds)	Calorie needs	Weight (Pounds)	Caloric needs
2	19.0	1365	19.0	1370	19.0	1376
3	34.0	1919	35.0	2039	36.0	2160
4	44.0	2080	46.0	2158	49.0	2277
6	57.0	1959	62.0	2118	66.0	2277
9	69.0	1960	75.0	2118	82.0	2277
12	81.0	2239	88.0	2415	96.0	2591
Adult	100.0	2184	110.0	2346	120.0	2504

	Estimated Adult Body Weight					
	130 Pounds		140 Pounds		150 Pounds	
Age (Months)	Weight (Pounds)	Caloric needs	Weight (Pounds)	Calorie needs	Weight (Pounds)	Caloric needs
2	19.0	1370	20.0	1370	21.0	1405
3	37.0	2257	39.0	2039	42.0	2507
4	51.0	2376	55.0	2158	59.0	2661
6	71.0	2455	76.0	2118	81.0	2699
9	88.0	2455	94.0	2118	101.0	2699
12	104.0	2811	111.0	2415	119.0	3085
Adult	130.0	2660	140.0	2346	150.0	2961

	Estimated Adult Body Weight			
	160 Pounds		175 Pounds	
Age (Months)	Weight (Pounds)	Caloric needs	Weight (Pounds)	Calorie needs
2	22.0	1458	25.0	1584
3	45.0	2649	48.0	2811
4	63.0	2802	67.0	2969
6	86.0	2879	93.0	3049
9	107.0	2841	116.0	3049
12	107.0	3225	137.0	3484
Adult	160.0	3108	175.0	3324

Source: Data are calculated from studies by A.L. Rainbird, H. Meyer, et al.

important to judge how much to feed by an additional evaluation of the puppy's appearance. Judge the amount to feed by the animal's weight and fat content.

> *The puppy should look trim with only a slight layer of fat over the ribs. The puppy is too fat if the ribs cannot be felt with gentle pressure on the rib cage. The puppy is too thin if the ribs can be easily seen as the puppy moves. If too fat, or too thin, regulate the diet until the puppy is in good condition. The desired condition varies with certain breeds— some tend to be more solid, others more trim.*
>
> *Emphasis should be placed on adjusting the diet every week to obtain the desired rate of growth, coat, body conformation, and spontaneous activity in the puppy, under the eye and hand of the owner.[7]*

A puppy's dietary intake should be examined and adjusted every week for its desired rate of growth, coat, body conformation, spontaneous activity, and most importantly prevention of orthopedic problems.

The information on overnutrition causing many medical problems is recent. In the past veterinarians were very happy to see owners bring in well-fed puppies of any breed. Owners were instructed and encouraged to feed their puppies so they would look as "healthy" as possible. Healthy meant, most importantly, that they were not thin. This is the wrong approach to counseling dog owners on care of their puppies, especially if they will mature to a large size.

Now it is well known that owners must learn to moderate energy intake in growing dogs (especially of the larger breeds). Periodic weight monitoring and control are essential. Maximal growth is not necessarily compatible with optimal growth. If owners continue to feed puppies so they can be proud of their animals' size, many problems can be expected. Rapid growth leads to abnormal skeletal development. Slower growth reduces the incidence of abnormalities and does not affect a dog's ability to eventually attain its normal adult size. The goal of feeding is to provide all the essential nutrients but while keeping the growing puppy "lean."

■ Evaluating Growth Rate in a Dog

In addition to evaluating a dog's nutritional condition by examining how much fat it carries, its weight can be compared with a standard. Table 4.3 shows the expected weight gain during growth of different sizes of mature dogs. This figure can be used to determine how an animal is growing.

Determination of a Dog's Caloric Needs during Pregnancy and Lactation

Developing canine fetuses increase little in size during the first four weeks of pregnancy. Pregnant dogs should not be overfed during this time, or they will become obese. Caloric intake should increase during the last half of pregnancy, and the number of daily feedings should also increase.

During lactation, calories are necessary for maintenance and milk production. For milk production, caloric requirements can be three to

Table 4.3. Weight (in pounds) of different sizes of mature dogs during growth

Age in Months						
2	3	4	6	9	12	Maturity
4.43	6.2	7.3	8.8	9.9	11.0	11.0
6.4	9.7	11.9	15.2	18.0	20.5	22.0
8.8	13.6	16.9	21.6	25.5	29.0	33.0
11.0	16.7	21.1	26.8	32.1	36.5	44.0
13.2	20.7	26.2	33.2	39.6	45.3	55.0
15.2	24.9	31.5	40.0	47.5	54.6	66.0
16.9	28.6	36.3	46.2	54.8	63.1	77.0
17.6	30.8	39.6	51.0	61.6	71.3	88.0
18.3	33.7	43.6	56.5	68.2	80.3	99.0
18.5	35.2	46.2	61.6	74.8	88.0	110.0
18.7	36.3	49.7	66.7	82.3	96.8	121.0
18.7	37.0	51.5	71.3	88.4	104.3	132.0
20.0	40.0	55.9	77.2	95.9	113.1	143.0
21.6	43.1	60.0	83.2	103.2	121.7	154.0
23.1	46.2	64.5	89.1	110.7	130.5	165.0
24.6	47.5	66.9	93.3	116.2	137.3	176.0

Source: Adapted from studies by H. Meyer.

five times greater than for maintenance. Lactating animals should eat three to four times a day.

Animals' weights should be optimum, and their diets should be complete and balanced at the time of breeding. Animals too thin at breeding may be in poor condition at weaning, and an obese animal may have a difficult delivery. The formula for estimating caloric requirements during pregnancy and lactation is based on optimum adult weight rather than actual weight. This allows thin animals to gain and obese ones to lose weight during pregnancy. The animal with an optimum adult body weight at breeding should weigh the same at weaning. Use the following formulas:

$$\text{Body weight}^{0.75} \times 132 = \text{Kilocalories needed for} \atop \text{pregnancy weeks 1–4} \tag{4.5}$$

$$\text{Pregnancy week 5} = \text{Maintenance kilocalories} \times 1.1 \tag{4.6}$$

$$\text{Pregnancy week 6–9} = \text{Maintenance kilocalories} \times 1.2 \tag{4.7}$$

$$\text{Lactation week 1} = \text{Maintenance kilocalories} \times 1.5 \tag{4.8}$$

$$\text{Lactation week 2} = \text{Maintenance kilocalories} \times 2 \tag{4.9}$$

$$\text{Lactation week 3–5} = \text{Maintenance kilocalories} \times 3 \tag{4.10}$$

Figures for maintenance body weight$^{0.75} \times 125$ can be found for any animal in Table 4.1. This value by can be increased by 5 to 6 percent to satisfy the needs of the formula for the first five weeks of pregnancy.

Determination of a Cat's Caloric Needs

Determination of energy requirements are easier for cats than dogs because body size of cats varies little. Instead of the complicated formula used to adjust for body surface area in dogs, adult cats are fed 70 to 80 kilocalories/kilogram of body weight. Active cats and cats living outside are fed the greater amount. During growth, pregnancy, and lactation, cats' energy needs increase to a degree comparable to dogs' in the same physiological state. Increases in nonfat tissues use about five kilocalories to produce a gram of new tissue. The daily caloric needs of a cat under different conditions are found in Table 4.4.

Table 4.4 Daily caloric requirements for cats

Indoor		Outdoor		Growing		Pregnancy		Lactation	
lb	kcal	lb	kcal	lb	kcal	lb	kcal	lb	kcal
4.0	127	4.0	145	1.0	141	4.0	182	4.0	455
4.5	143	4.5	164	1.5	192	4.5	205	4.5	511
5.0	159	5.0	159	2.0	231	5.0	227	5.0	568
5.5	175	5.5	200	2.5	260	5.5	250	5.5	625
6.0	191	6.0	218	3.0	281	6.0	273	6.0	682
6.5	207	6.5	236	3.5	294	6.5	295	6.5	739
7.0	223	7.0	255	4.0	302	7.0	318	7.0	795
7.5	239	7.5	273	4.5	305	7.5	341	7.5	852
8.0	254	8.0	291	5.0	307	8.0	364	8.0	909
8.5	270	8.5	309	5.5	305	8.5	386	8.5	966
9.0	286	9.0	327	6.0	300	9.0	409	9.0	1023
9.5	302	9.5	345	6.5	298	9.5	432	9.5	1080
10.0	318	10.0	364	7.0	299	10.0	455	10.0	1136
10.5	334	10.5	382	7.5	303	10.5	477	10.5	1193
11.0	350	11.0	400	8.0	312	11.0	500	11.0	1250
11.5	366	11.5	418	8.5	324	11.5	523	11.5	1307
12.0	382	12.0	436	9.0	343	12.0	545	12.0	1364

Source: Data are calculated from NRC recommendations.

Controlling a Pet's Energy Intake

Pet food manufacturers advise pet owners to not feed owner-prepared foods. They give many reasons such as these foods adversely affect a pet's health. They also claim owner-prepared foods are more likely to result in overeating and obesity. Pet food manufacturers are correct in claiming that mixing and feeding table scraps with dog food results in overeating and obesity. This also happens when mixing canned pet foods and dry foods, one of the pet food industry's recommendations. Anything enhancing palatability results in a pet eating too much.

If human-prepared foods are fed separately, in amounts too small to meet an animal's energy needs, and in addition a dry food is fed free-choice, the pet is not likely to overeat. The pet may eat less dry food than it needs because it has the chance to eat a more palatable human food. Feeding this combination without mixing them is an acceptable way to feed pets.

Formulating and Feeding Owner-Prepared Diets

Pet owners have no control over the formulation of commercial pet foods. Caloric consumption with these foods is merely an estimate. All of the owner-prepared diets in this book list the caloric content. The tables in this chapter give a pet's caloric requirements and can be used for finding how much of any diet to feed. The caloric content of any food is determined by the digestibility of its ingredients. Owner-prepared diets in this book contain highly digestible ingredients, making their caloric content more completely available.

Formulating a pet's diet, the preparer has control over the selection and use of every ingredient it will contain. That allows formulation of a diet with a known caloric content.

References

1. Finke, Mark D. 1991. Evaluation of the energy requirements of adult kennel dogs. *Journal of Nutrition* 121:S22–S28.

2. Kienzle, Ellen and Anna Rainbird. 1991. Maintenance energy requirement of dogs: What is the correct value for the calculation of metabolic body weight in dogs? *Journal of Nutrition.* 121:S39–S40.

3. Kronfeld, David S. 1973. Diet and the performance of racing sled dogs. *Journal of the American Veterinary Medical Association* 162:470–473.

4. Burger, I.H. 1993. A basic guide to nutrient requirements. In *The Waltham Book of Companion Animal Nutrition,* edited by I.H. Burger, 5–24. Oxford: Pergamon Press.

5. Alpo Advisory Board. 1984. *Canine Nutrition and Feeding Management,* 29. Lehigh Valley, Pa.: ALPO Pet Center.

6. Rainbird, Anna L. 1987. Growth and energy requirements of dogs. In *Nutrition, Malnutrition and Dietetics in the Dog and Cat,* Proceedings, international symposium, 44–45. London: British Veterinary Association.

7. Alpo Advisory Board. 1984. *Canine Nutrition and Feeding Management,* 39. Lehigh Valley, Pa.: ALPO Pet Center.

CHAPTER 5
Feeding a Normal Dog or Cat

Owners can prepare diets for their pets with no more difficulty than for their own needs. The following diets contain foods that humans commonly use for their own diets. This chapter provides recipes for feeding adult dogs and cats a maintenance diet. Also included are diets for growing puppies and kittens. Some very active or hardworking dogs require greater amounts of energy than growing animals. Recipes are given to sustain the needs of such animals.

Preparing Diets

Unless stated, the following diets are all nutritionally balanced and complete. Each recipe lists quantities of proteins and fats that cannot be compared with those listed for commercial pet foods. Commercial products contain higher concentrations of proteins. These foods have higher levels because digestibility and availability for their proteins are poor compared with those in owner-prepared recipes. Commercial pet foods need up to twice as much protein as owner-prepared diets because it takes that much to supply amino acid requirements. The amino acid content of owner-prepared diets is also closer to ideal so that less protein is needed to provide for an animal's needs.

Fat content varies with each diet. In many recipes vegetable oil is the primary source of fat. If a pet gains weight and its body fat exceeds the ideal, dietary oil is reduced. Most diets contain other sources of fat that provide essential unsaturated fatty acids, so eliminating vegetable oil will not result in a deficiency.

The diets contain more than required amounts of sodium chloride but much less than commercial pet foods, which contain approximately 1 percent salt. Iodized table salt can be used to add flavor if desired.

■ Vegetable Supplements

To each of the following diets, vegetables can be added. They are not necessary to make a diet nutritionally complete. The number of calories added with the inclusion of vegetables can be found in Table 5.1. Uncooked vegetables contain few available calories. If they are included or fed as snacks, it is not necessary to calculate their caloric contribution to the pet's intake. They provide additional fiber.

■ Vitamin and Mineral Supplementation[1]

When the diet cannot be balanced with natural foods to provide vitamin and mineral requirements, it is necessary to supplement with a vitamin-mineral preparation. Supplements prepared for pets are used

Table 5.1. Caloric content of vegetable portions

Vegetable	Quantity	Kilocalories
Asparagus, cooked	½ cup	22
Broccoli, cooked	½ cup	23
Brussels sprouts, cooked	½ cup	30
Cabbage, cooked	½ cup	16
Carrots, cooked	½ cup	35
Celery, cooked	½ cup	11
Green beans, cooked	½ cup	22
Peas, green, cooked	½ cup	67
Peppers, sweet, cooked	½ cup	12
Spinach, cooked	½ cup	1
Squash, summer, cooked	½ cup	18
Tomato, cooked	½ cup	30
Turnip, cooked	½ cup	14

Source: Bowes and Church's Food Values of Portions Commonly Used.

unless they are not tolerated. The most common supplements prepared for pets contain flavoring agents, binders, fillers, and other additives that can cause gastrointestinal problems in animals with allergies. Such additives are less likely to be used in supplements prepared for humans.

The amount of vitamin and mineral supplement to give is based on an animal's caloric intake or body weight. Supplements formulated for an adult human meet the average needs for a person weighing much more than most dogs. Thus, a vitamin-mineral tablet for a human contains concentrations of ingredients too high for most dogs. Some may believe that excessive amounts of vitamins and minerals are not harmful, that more is better than the required amounts. Excessive amounts of most vitamins and minerals are not harmful.

An excess amount of vitamin A or D is harmful, however. Excess vitamin A is toxic to the liver, especially when a toxin is present or the liver must detoxify a chemical (drug). Excess vitamin D is also toxic in that it stimulates absorption of excess calcium.

Excess dietary copper causes large amounts to accumulate in the liver. If the liver is unable to excrete copper, it can cause severe liver damage.

Vitamin supplementation is based on caloric consumption. Each 1000 kilocalories of food should contain a certain level of each vitamin. The recommendations are more precise for growing animals than for adults. All of the diets in this book contain vitamins at levels based on the caloric content. It is not necessary to supplement any of these diets with vitamins unless the recipes state that a supplement is required.

It is also possible to make vitamin recommendations based on an animal's body weight. Tables 5.2 and 5.3 gives vitamin recommendations based on an animal's weight. Table 5.3 gives adjustments for using human vitamin-mineral preparations based on an animal's size. Although a growing animal has greater requirements than an adult, the vitamin content based on amounts per 1000 kilocalories is almost the same for growing and adult animals. The growing animal receives more vitamins because it eats more per pound body weight. Cooking destroys vitamins, so vitamin supplements are added after cooking and before feeding.

Vitamin-mineral supplements are formulated for small animals so they meet the needs for their varying body size. Examples include PET-TABS® and VI-SORBITS® made by SmithKline Beecham. The former contains ingredients such as liver (beef and pork), fish meal, wheat germ meal, and a number of other additives and fillers that could cause problems in animals with gastrointestinal problems. If

Table 5.2. Vitamin requirements for growing and adult cats and dogs
(amounts per kilogram body weight per day)

Vitamin	Growing Cat	Adult Cat	Growing Dog	Adult Dog
A	200 IU	75 IU	202 IU	75 IU
D	20 IU	8 IU	22 IU	8 IU
E	1.2 IU	0.5 IU	1.2 IU	0.5 IU
K[a]	2 μg	2 μg	2 μg	2 μg
Thiamin	200 μg	200 μg	54 μg	20 μg
Riboflavin	160 μg	160 μg	100 μg	50 μg
Pantothenate	200 μg	200 μg	400 μg	200 μg
Niacin	1600 μg	1600 μg	450 μg	225 μg
Pyridoxine	160 μg	160 μg	60 μg	22 μg
Folic acid	32 μg	32 μg	8 μg	4 μg
Biotin	2.8 μg	2.8 μg	—	—
B_{12}	0.8 μg	0.8 μg	1 μg	0.5 μg
Choline	96 mg	96 mg	50 mg	25 mg

Source: NRC requirements for cats and dogs.

[a]The diet does not need to provide this vitamin unless an animal is being given antibiotics or antivitamin compounds for an extended period.

these are tolerated, they can be given more easily than human vitamin-mineral preparations. The animal preparations are not regulated as closely by governmental agencies for such things as potency. For animals with food intolerances and allergies, human nonallergenic preparations can be given, and the amount to use in any diet is one-fifth of a capsule or tablet for each tablet of pet vitamin-mineral tablet called for in a recipe. An example of a nonallergenic human preparation is a multiple vitamin-mineral product made by Nature's Way Products, Springville, Utah.

Diets for dogs not containing sardines lack vitamin B_{12}, even with a vitamin-mineral supplement. Sardines are added to provide vitamin B_{12}, which can also be added by including liver in the diet. One reason

Table 5.3. Percent of adult human vitamin-mineral capsule to give
a dog daily

Dog's Body Weight in Pounds									
15	30	45	60	75	90	105	120	135	150
10%	20%	30%	40%	50%	60%	70%	80%	90%	100%

for not using liver is that it contains very high levels of vitamin A and sometimes excess vitamin D. Excess of either vitamin is toxic. Thus, liver should not be given daily to a dog or cat. Sardines also increase palatability as some diets lack flavor. If sardines are not fed, vitamin B_{12} tablets can be added. (Removing 2 tablespoons sardines from a diet lowers the caloric content by 68 kilocalories, protein content by 6.2 grams, and fat by 4.6 grams.) Most tablets contain 1000 micrograms, which is 50 times more than a dog requires. It is probably not necessary to give this vitamin more than once a week. Many dogs and cats eat diets very deficient in vitamin B_{12} for months and sometimes for years without signs of vitamin B_{12} deficiency. Thus, it is not important to supplement owner-prepared diets with additional vitamin B_{12}.

Mineral supplementation is based on the number of calories consumed. Each 1000 kilocalories of pet food should contain a certain level of each mineral. The recommendations are more precise for growing animals than for adults. Each of the diets in this book contains minerals at levels based on its caloric content. None need to be supplemented with minerals unless a recipe states that a supplement is required. It is also possible to make mineral recommendations based on an animal's body weight (Table 5.4). A growing animals has greater requirements than an adult. The mineral content based on amounts per 1000 kilocalories is almost the same for growing and adult animals. The growing animals gets more minerals because it eats more per pound body weight. Bonemeal provides a balanced ratio of calcium to phosphorus and provides trace minerals. Bonemeal is provided in the recipes as tablets. An equivalent amount can be provided as powder. One bonemeal tablet is equivalent to a level one-fourth teaspoon of bonemeal powder. (Measurement of one level portion of a teaspoon can be made with a measuring spoon and does not involve decisions on how much is a "rounded teaspoon." I made this calculation using Solgar's Bone Meal Powder with vitamin B_{12}. Solgar's web site (*www.solgar.com*) has a comprehensive list of retail sources readily available throughout the country.

■ Determination of Caloric Needs

Determine a pet's ideal body weight. Refer to Tables 4.1, 4.2, or 4.4 on caloric requirements in Chapter 4 to find the number of calories to feed each day. The following recipes show how to prepare an amount with a specific caloric content. That amount is appropriate for an adult pet at a certain weight. If the size of the recipe is inappropriate for any animal, reduce or increase it to meet the pet's nutritional needs.

Table 5.4. Mineral requirements for growing and adult cats and dogs (minimum amounts per kilogram body weight per day)

Mineral	Growing Cat	Adult Cat	Growing Dog	Adult Dog
Calcium	400 mg	128 mg	320 mg	119 mg
Phosphorus	300 mg	96 mg	240 mg	89 mg
Sodium	25 mg	8 mg	30 mg	11 mg
Potassium	200 mg	64 mg	240 mg	89 mg
Chloride	95 mg	30 mg	46 mg	17 mg
Magnesium	20 mg	6.4 mg	22 mg	8 mg
Iron	4 mg	1.28 mg	1.74 mg	0.65 mg
Copper	0.25 mg	0.08 mg	0.16 mg	0.06 mg
Manganese	0.25 mg	0.08 mg	0.28 mg	0.10 mg
Zinc	2.5 mg	0.8 mg	1.94 mg	0.72 mg
Iodine	0.017 mg	0.006 mg	0.032 mg	0.012 mg
Selenium	5 µg	1.6 µg	6 µg	2.2 µg

Source: NRC requirements for cats and dogs.

Diets for Adult Dogs

Eggs and Rice Diet

3 eggs, large, hard-boiled

2 cups rice, long-grain, cooked

2 tablespoons sardines, canned, tomato sauce

2 tablespoons vegetable (canola) oil

¼ teaspoon salt substitute—potassium chloride

4 bonemeal tablets (10-grain or equivalent)

1 multiple vitamin-mineral tablet

Provides 964 kilocalories, 34.1 grams protein, 49.4 grams fat
Supports caloric needs of a 33- to 34-pound dog
This diet is relatively high in fat and is suitable for an active or working dog. To modify this diet for less active dogs, the vegetable oil can be omitted, which reduces the caloric content

to about 712 kilocalories. Without the vegetable oil the bone-meal tablets can be reduced to three.

Omission of sardines reduces caloric content by 68 kilocalories, protein by 6.2 grams, and fat by 4.6 grams.

Eggs and Potato Diet

3 eggs, large, hard-boiled

3 cups potato, cooked with skin

2 tablespoons sardines, canned, tomato sauce

¼ teaspoon salt substitute—potassium chloride

4 bonemeal tablets (10-grain or equivalent)

1 multiple vitamin-mineral tablet

Provides 708 kilocalories, 34.5 grams protein, 21 grams fat
Supports caloric needs of a 22-pound dog
Omission of sardines reduces caloric content by 68 kilocalories, protein by 6.2 grams, and fat by 4.6 grams.

Eggs and Macaroni Diet

3 eggs, large, hard-boiled

2 cups macaroni, cooked

2 tablespoons sardines, canned, tomato sauce

¼ teaspoon salt substitute—potassium chloride

¹⁄₁₀ teaspoon table salt

4 bonemeal tablets (10-grain or equivalent)

1 multiple vitamin-mineral tablet

Provides 696 kilocalories, 39.1 grams protein, 22.4 grams fat
Supports caloric needs of a 22-pound dog
Omission of sardines reduces caloric content by 68 kilocalories, protein by 6.2 grams, and fat by 4.6 grams.

Cottage Cheese and Rice Diet

1 cup cottage cheese, 2 percent fat

2¹/₂ cups rice, long-grain, cooked

2 tablespoons sardines, canned, tomato sauce

1¹/₂ tablespoons vegetable (canola) oil

¹/₄ teaspoon salt substitute—potassium chloride

4 bonemeal tablets (10-grain or equivalent)

1 multiple vitamin-mineral tablet

Provides 973 kilocalories, 47.8 grams protein, 31.2 grams fat
Supports caloric needs of a 34-pound dog
Diets containing cottage cheese are much higher in sodium; water consumption will be greater on these diets than on others.

Omission of sardines reduces caloric content by 68 kilocalories, protein by 6.2 grams, and fat by 4.6 grams.

Cottage Cheese and Potato Diet

²/₃ cup cottage cheese, 2 percent fat

2 cups potato, cooked with skin

2 tablespoons sardines, canned, tomato sauce

1¹/₂ tablespoons vegetable (canola) oil

¹/₄ teaspoon salt substitute—potassium chloride

4 bonemeal tablets (10-grain or equivalent)

1 multiple vitamin-mineral tablet

Provides 661 kilocalories, 32.7 grams protein, 28.8 grams fat
Supports caloric needs of a 20- to 21-pound dog
Omission of sardines reduces caloric content by 68 kilocalories, protein by 6.2 grams, and fat by 4.6 grams.

Cottage Cheese and Macaroni Diet

⅔ *cup cottage cheese, 2 percent fat*

2½ *cups macaroni, cooked*

2 *tablespoons sardines, canned, tomato sauce*

2 *tablespoons vegetable (canola) oil*

¼ *teaspoon salt substitute—potassium chloride*

4 *bonemeal tablets (10-grain or equivalent)*

1 *multiple vitamin-mineral tablet*

Provides 946 kilocalories, 43.6 grams protein, 37.9 grams fat
Supports caloric needs of a 33-pound dog
Omission of sardines reduces caloric content by 68 kilocalories, protein by 6.2 grams, and fat by 4.6 grams.

Poultry Meat and Rice Diet

⅓ *pound poultry meat (raw weight), cooked*

2 *cups rice, long-grain, cooked*

2 *tablespoons sardines, canned, tomato sauce*

1 *tablespoon vegetable (canola) oil*

¼ *teaspoon salt substitute—potassium chloride*

1/10 *teaspoon table salt*

4 *bonemeal tablets (10-grain or equivalent)*

1 *multiple vitamin-mineral tablet*

Provides 879 kilocalories, 43.1 grams protein, 37.3 grams fat
Supports caloric needs of a 29- to 30-pound dog
Omission of sardines reduces caloric content by 68 kilocalories, protein by 6.2 grams, and fat by 4.6 grams.

Poultry Meat and Potato Diet

⅓ pound poultry meat (raw weight), cooked

3 cups potato, cooked with skin

2 tablespoons sardines, canned, tomato sauce

1 tablespoon vegetable (canola) oil

¼ teaspoon salt substitute—potassium chloride

¹/₁₀ teaspoon table salt

4 bonemeal tablets (10-grain or equivalent)

1 multiple vitamin-mineral tablet

Provides 851 kilocalories, 42.4 grams protein, 34.3 grams fat
Supports caloric needs of a 28- to 29-pound dog
Omission of sardines reduces caloric content by 68 kilocalories, protein by 6.2 grams, and fat by 4.6 grams.

Poultry Meat and Macaroni Diet

⅓ pound poultry meat (raw weight), cooked

2 cups macaroni, cooked

2 tablespoons sardines, canned, tomato sauce

1 tablespoon vegetable (canola) oil

¼ teaspoon salt substitute—potassium chloride

4 bonemeal tablets (10-grain or equivalent)

1 multiple vitamin-mineral tablet

Provides 940 kilocalories, 50.4 grams protein, 36.2 grams fat
Supports caloric needs of a 32- to 33-pound dog
Omission of sardines reduces caloric content by 68 kilocalories, protein by 6.2 grams, and fat by 4.6 grams.

Beef Meat and Rice Diet

⅓ pound very lean beef (raw weight), cooked

2 cups rice, long-grain, cooked

2 tablespoons sardines, canned, tomato sauce

1 tablespoon vegetable (canola) oil

¼ teaspoon salt substitute—potassium chloride

5 bonemeal tablets (10-grain or equivalent)

1 multiple vitamin-mineral tablet

Provides 890 kilocalories, 44.3 grams protein, 38.1 grams fat
Supports caloric needs of a 30-pound dog
Omission of sardines reduces caloric content by 68 kilocalories, protein by 6.2 grams, and fat by 4.6 grams.

Beef Meat and Potato Diet

⅓ pound very lean beef (raw weight), cooked

3 cups potato, cooked with skin

2 tablespoons sardines, canned, tomato sauce

1 tablespoon vegetable (canola) oil

5 bonemeal tablets (10-grain or equivalent)

1 multiple vitamin-mineral tablet

Provides 862 kilocalories, 43.6 grams protein, 35.1 grams fat
Supports caloric needs of a 29-pound dog
Omission of sardines reduces caloric content by 68 kilocalories, protein by 6.2 grams, and fat by 4.6 grams.

Beef Meat and Macaroni Diet

⅓ pound very lean beef (raw weight), cooked

2 cups macaroni, cooked

2 tablespoons sardines, canned, tomato sauce

1 tablespoon vegetable (canola) oil

5 bonemeal tablets (10-grain or equivalent)

1 multiple vitamin-mineral tablet

Provides 951 kilocalories, 51.2 grams protein, 37.1 grams fat
Supports caloric needs of a 33-pound dog
Omission of sardines reduces caloric content by 68 kilocalories, protein by 6.2 grams, and fat by 4.6 grams.

It is possible to substitute other pastas for macaroni without changing the nutrients provided. In comparing the preceding diets, feeding macaroni provides a medium size dog 8 grams of protein more than rice or potato. However, the digestibility of macaroni is poorer than for rice or potato.

Vegetarian Diets for Adult Dogs

Completely balanced vegetarian diets can be fed to dogs without fear of causing any nutritional deficiency. The digestibility of vegetable proteins is less complete than for proteins of animal origin. Vegetarian diets are usually less expensive than those containing animal protein. These diets require supplementation with vitamin B_{12}, a vitamin found only in food prepared from animal sources. This vitamin can be given once a week.

Tofu and Rice Diet

⅔ cup tofu, raw firm

2 cups rice, long-grain, cooked

¼ teaspoon salt substitute—potassium chloride

¹/₁₀ teaspoon table salt

3 bonemeal tablets (10-grain or equivalent)

1 multiple vitamin-mineral tablet

(vitamin B₁₂ once a week)

Provides 679 kilocalories, 36.6 grams protein, 18.4 grams fat
Supports caloric needs of a 21-pound dog

Tofu and Potato Diet

½ cup tofu, raw firm

2 cups potato, cooked with skin

¹/₁₀ teaspoon table salt

2 bonemeal tablets (10-grain or equivalent)

1 multiple vitamin-mineral tablet

(vitamin B₁₂ once a week)

Provides 455 kilocalories, 25.9 grams protein, 11.3 grams fat
Supports caloric needs of a 12- to 13-pound dog

Tofu and Macaroni Diet

$\frac{1}{2}$ *cup tofu, raw firm*

2 cups macaroni, cooked

1 teaspoon vegetable (canola) oil

$\frac{1}{4}$ *teaspoon salt substitute—potassium chloride*

$\frac{1}{10}$ *teaspoon table salt*

4 bonemeal tablets (10-grain or equivalent)

1 multiple vitamin-mineral tablet

(vitamin B$_{12}$ once a week)

Provides 721 kilocalories, 36.6 grams protein, 18.4 grams fat
Supports caloric needs of a 23-pound dog

Tofu, Lentils, and Potato Diet

$\frac{1}{2}$ *cup tofu, raw firm*

1 cup lentils, boiled

2 cups potato, cooked with skin

2 teaspoons vegetable (canola) oil

$\frac{1}{10}$ *teaspoon table salt*

4 bonemeal tablets (10-grain or equivalent)

1 multiple vitamin-mineral tablet

(vitamin B$_{12}$ once a week)

Provides 775 kilocalories, 43.9 grams protein, 22 grams fat
Supports caloric needs of a 25-pound dog

Tofu, Lentils, and Rice Diet

1/4 cup tofu, raw firm

1 cup lentils, boiled

1 cup rice, long-grain, cooked

2 teaspoons vegetable (canola) oil

1/4 teaspoon salt substitute—potassium chloride

1/10 teaspoon table salt

4 bonemeal tablets (10-grain or equivalent)

1 multiple vitamin-mineral tablet

(vitamin B$_{12}$ once a week)

Provides 629 kilocalories, 33 grams protein, 18 grams fat
Supports caloric needs of a 19-pound dog

Tofu, Lentils, and Macaroni Diet

1/4 cup tofu, raw firm

1 cup lentils, boiled

2 cups macaroni, cooked

1 teaspoon vegetable (canola) oil

1/4 teaspoon salt substitute—potassium chloride

1/10 teaspoon table salt

5 bonemeal tablets (10-grain or equivalent)

1 multiple vitamin-mineral tablet

(vitamin B$_{12}$ once a week)

Provides 861 kilocalories, 44.6 grams protein, 13.6 grams fat
Supports caloric needs of a 29-pound dog

Tofu, Black-Eyed Peas, and Rice Diet

⅓ *cup tofu, raw firm*

1 cup black-eyed peas, boiled

1 cup rice, long-grain, cooked

2 teaspoons vegetable (canola) oil

¼ *teaspoon salt substitute—potassium chloride*

¹⁄₁₀ *teaspoon table salt*

3 bonemeal tablets (10-grain or equivalent)

1 multiple vitamin-mineral tablet

(vitamin B$_{12}$ once a week)

Provides 627 kilocalories, 31.7 grams protein, 19.1 grams fat
Supports caloric needs of a 19-pound dog

Soybean and Rice Diet

1 cup soybeans, mature, boiled

2 cups rice, long-grain, cooked

¼ *teaspoon salt substitute—potassium chloride*

¹⁄₁₀ *teaspoon table salt*

4 bonemeal tablets (10-grain or equivalent)

1 multiple vitamin-mineral tablet

(vitamin B$_{12}$ once a week)

Provides 733 kilocalories, 38.7 grams protein, 19 grams fat
Supports caloric needs of a 23- to 24-pound dog

Soybean and Potato Diet

1 cup soybeans, mature, boiled

2 cups potato, cooked with skin

$\frac{1}{10}$ teaspoon table salt

3 bonemeal tablets (10-grain or equivalent)

1 multiple vitamin-mineral tablet

(vitamin B$_{12}$ once a week)

Provides 570 kilocalories, 34.6 grams protein, 15.7 grams fat
Supports caloric needs of a 17-pound dog

Soybean and Macaroni Diet

1 cup soybeans, mature, boiled

2 cups macaroni, cooked

$\frac{1}{4}$ teaspoon salt substitute—potassium chloride

$\frac{1}{10}$ teaspoon table salt

5 bonemeal tablets (10-grain or equivalent)

1 multiple vitamin-mineral tablet

(vitamin B$_{12}$ once a week)

Provides 792 kilocalories, 45.3 grams protein, 17.8 grams fat
Supports caloric needs of a 26-pound dog

Diets for Growing Dogs

Growth requires greater amounts of protein, calories, vitamins, and minerals. Puppies can double their body weight in a short time. A number of recipes follow that are based on using animal sources of proteins. It is possible to support a puppy's growth by feeding a vegetarian diet, and recipes are included. Because vegetable and cereal proteins are not as well digested as animal proteins, vegetarian diets need greater amounts of proteins than diets based on animal proteins.

Beef Meat and Rice Diet

½ pound very lean beef (raw weight), cooked

1½ cups rice, long-grain, cooked

2 tablespoons sardines, canned, tomato sauce

1 teaspoon vegetable (canola) oil

¼ teaspoon salt substitute—potassium chloride

⅒ teaspoon table salt

5 bonemeal tablets (10-grain or equivalent)

1 multiple vitamin-mineral tablet

Provides 815 kilocalories, 54.6 grams protein, 34.3 grams fat
See Table 4.2 in Chapter 4 for a puppy's caloric needs.
Omission of sardines reduces caloric content by 68 kilocalories, protein by 6.2 grams, and fat by 4.6 grams.

Beef Meat and Potato Diet

½ pound very lean beef (raw weight), cooked

2½ cups potato, cooked with skin

2 tablespoons sardines, canned, tomato sauce

1 tablespoon vegetable (canola) oil

¼ teaspoon salt substitute—potassium chloride

1/10 teaspoon table salt

6 bonemeal tablets (10-grain or equivalent)

1 multiple vitamin-mineral tablet

Provides 858 kilocalories, 51.2 grams protein, 29.7 grams fat
See Table 4.2 in Chapter 4 for a puppy's caloric needs.
Omission of sardines reduces caloric content by 68 kilocalories, protein by 6.2 grams, and fat by 4.6 grams.

Beef Meat and Macaroni Diet

½ pound very lean beef (raw weight), cooked

2½ cups macaroni, cooked

2 tablespoons sardines, canned, tomato sauce

1 tablespoon vegetable (canola) oil

½ teaspoon salt substitute—potassium chloride

1/10 teaspoon table salt

7 bonemeal tablets (10-grain or equivalent)

1 multiple vitamin-mineral tablet

Provides 1081 kilocalories, 64.9 grams protein, 45 grams fat
See Table 4.2 in Chapter 4 for a puppy's caloric needs.
Omission of sardines reduces caloric content by 68 kilocalories, protein by 6.2 grams, and fat by 4.6 grams.

Eggs and Rice Diet

5 eggs, large, hard-boiled

1½ cups rice, long-grain, cooked

2 tablespoons sardines, canned, tomato sauce

⅓ teaspoon salt substitute—potassium chloride

4 bonemeal tablets (10-grain or equivalent)

1 multiple vitamin-mineral tablet

Provides 765 kilocalories, 44.5 grams protein, 32 grams fat
See Table 4.2 in Chapter 4 for a puppy's caloric needs.
Omission of sardines reduces caloric content by 68 kilocalories, protein by 6.2 grams, and fat by 4.6 grams.

Eggs and Potato Diet

5 eggs, large, hard-boiled

2½ cups potato, cooked with skin

2 tablespoons sardines, canned, tomato sauce

¼ teaspoon salt substitute—potassium chloride

4 bonemeal tablets (10-grain or equivalent)

1 multiple vitamin-mineral tablet

Provides 798 kilocalories, 45.5 grams protein, 31.7 grams fat
See Table 4.2 in Chapter 4 for a puppy's caloric needs.
Omission of sardines reduces caloric content by 68 kilocalories, protein by 6.2 grams, and fat by 4.6 grams.

Eggs and Macaroni Diet

5 eggs, large, hard-boiled

2½ cups macaroni, cooked

2 tablespoons sardines, canned, tomato sauce

⅓ teaspoon salt substitute—potassium chloride

5 bonemeal tablets (10-grain or equivalent)

1 multiple vitamin-mineral tablet

Provides 952 kilocalories, 54.6 grams protein, 33.6 grams fat
See Table 4.2 in Chapter 4 for a puppy's caloric needs.
Omission of sardines reduces caloric content by 68 kilocalories, protein by 6.2 grams, and fat by 4.6 grams.

Poultry Meat and Rice Diet

½ pound poultry meat (raw weight), cooked

2 cups rice, long-grain, cooked

2 tablespoons sardines, canned, tomato sauce

1 teaspoon vegetable (canola) oil

⅓ teaspoon salt substitute—potassium chloride

⅒ teaspoon table salt

6 bonemeal tablets (10-grain or equivalent)

1 multiple vitamin-mineral tablet

Provides 929 kilocalories, 56.5 grams protein, 35.9 grams fat
See Table 4.2 in Chapter 4 for a puppy's caloric needs.
Omission of sardines reduces caloric content by 68 kilocalories, protein by 6.2 grams, and fat by 4.6 grams.

Poultry Meat and Potato Diet

½ pound poultry meat (raw weight), cooked

3 cups potato, cooked with skin

2 tablespoons sardines, canned, tomato sauce

1 teaspoon vegetable (canola) oil

¼ teaspoon salt substitute—potassium chloride

¹/₁₀ teaspoon table salt

6 bonemeal tablets (10-grain or equivalent)

1 multiple vitamin-mineral tablet

Provides 901 kilocalories, 55.1 grams protein, 32.9 grams fat
See Table 4.2 in Chapter 4 for a puppy's caloric needs.
Omission of sardines reduces caloric content by 68 kilocalories, protein by 6.2 grams, and fat by 4.6 grams.

Poultry Meat and Macaroni Diet

½ pound poultry meat (raw weight), cooked

2½ cups macaroni, cooked

2 tablespoons sardines, canned, tomato sauce

1 tablespoon vegetable (canola) oil

⅓ teaspoon salt substitute—potassium chloride

¹/₁₀ teaspoon table salt

7 bonemeal tablets (10-grain or equivalent)

1 multiple vitamin-mineral tablet

Provides 1065 kilocalories, 63.6 grams protein, 43.9 grams fat
See Table 4.2 in Chapter 4 for a puppy's caloric needs.
Omission of sardines reduces caloric content by 68 kilocalories, protein by 6.2 grams, and fat by 4.6 grams.

Cottage Cheese and Rice Diet

1½ cups cottage cheese, 2 percent fat

2½ cups rice, long-grain, cooked

2 tablespoons sardines, canned, tomato sauce

1 tablespoon vegetable (canola) oil

⅓ teaspoon salt substitute—potassium chloride

7 bonemeal tablets (10-grain or equivalent)

1 multiple vitamin-mineral tablet

Provides 1021 kilocalories, 64.6 grams protein, 26.5 grams fat

See Table 4.2 in Chapter 4 for a puppy's caloric needs.

Omission of sardines reduces caloric content by 68 kilocalories, protein by 6.2 grams, and fat by 4.6 grams.

Cottage Cheese and Potato Diet

1⅓ cups cottage cheese, 2 percent fat

2½ cups potato, cooked with skin

2 tablespoons sardines, canned, tomato sauce

2 tablespoons vegetable (canola) oil

¼ teaspoon salt substitute—potassium chloride

6 bonemeal tablets (10-grain or equivalent)

1 multiple vitamin-mineral tablet

Provides 936 kilocalories, 54.7 grams protein, 39 grams fat

See Table 4.2 in Chapter 4 for a puppy's caloric needs.

Omission of sardines reduces caloric content by 68 kilocalories, protein by 6.2 grams, and fat by 4.6 grams.

Cottage Cheese and Macaroni Diet

1¹/₃ cups cottage cheese, 2 percent fat

2¹/₂ cups macaroni, cooked

2 tablespoons sardines, canned, tomato sauce

2 tablespoons vegetable (canola) oil

¹/₃ teaspoon salt substitute—potassium chloride

7 bonemeal tablets (10-grain or equivalent)

1 multiple vitamin-mineral tablet

Provides 1124 kilocalories, 71.2 grams protein, 42 grams fat
See Table 4.2 in Chapter 4 for a puppy's caloric needs.
Omission of sardines reduces caloric content by 68 kilocalories, protein by 6.2 grams, and fat by 4.6 grams.

Vegetarian Diets for Growing Dogs

Soybean and Rice Diet

2 cups soybeans, mature, boiled

2 cups rice, long-grain, cooked

1 teaspoon vegetable (canola) oil

¹/₄ teaspoon salt substitute—potassium chloride

¹/₁₀ teaspoon table salt

6 bonemeal tablets (10-grain or equivalent)

1 multiple vitamin-mineral tablet

(vitamin B$_{12}$ once a week)

Provides 1078 kilocalories, 67.8 grams protein, 39.5 grams
fat
See Table 4.2 in Chapter 4 for a puppy's caloric needs.

Soybean and Potato Diet

2 cups soybeans, mature, boiled

2½ cups potato, cooked with skin

2 teaspoons vegetable (canola) oil

⅒ teaspoon table salt

6 bonemeal tablets (10-grain or equivalent)

1 multiple vitamin-mineral tablet

(vitamin B$_{12}$ once a week)

Provides 1028 kilocalories, 64.9 grams protein, 41.4 grams fat

See Table 4.2 in Chapter 4 for a puppy's caloric needs.

Tofu, Black-Eyed Peas, and Rice Diet

1 cup tofu, raw firm

1 cup black-eyed peas, boiled

1 cup rice, long-grain, cooked

1 teaspoon vegetable (canola) oil

¼ teaspoon salt substitute—potassium chloride

⅒ teaspoon table salt

4 bonemeal tablets (10-grain or equivalent)

1 multiple vitamin-mineral tablet

(vitamin B$_{12}$ once a week)

Provides 914 kilocalories, 58.5 grams protein, 39 grams fat

See Table 4.2 in Chapter 4 for a puppy's caloric needs.

All vegetarian diets must be supplemented with vitamin B$_{12}$. This vitamin is not found in foods that come from plant material.

Biscuits for Dogs

Wheat Flour, Wheat Germ, Brewer's Yeast

2 cups wheat flour, unbleached

½ cup wheat germ

½ cup brewer's yeast

3 tablespoons vegetable (canola) oil

1 cup chicken broth

⅙ teaspoon table salt

Flavoring, such as garlic powder

5 calcium carbonate tablets (2000 milligrams calcium)

Mix flour, wheat germ, brewer's yeast, and salt. Mix in oil and chicken broth (with added flavoring). Work dough into a one-half-inch-thick piece from which biscuits are prepared with biscuit or cookie cutter. Bake in preheated oven at 400°F for 20 to 25 minutes. Turn heat off and allow biscuits to dry for two hours. Store in refrigerator or freezer. Recipe contains 1773 kilocalories, 72.3 grams protein, and 51.6 grams fat. Recipe can make 36 biscuits containing 50 kilocalories, 2 grams protein, and 1.5 grams fat each.

Whole Wheat Flour, Cornmeal, Milk Powder

1 cup whole wheat flour

1 cup cornmeal

½ cup nonfat dry milk powder

4 tablespoons margarine (¼ cup)

½ cup bulgur, cooked

2 teaspoons baking powder

1 cup water

Flavoring, such as garlic powder

3 calcium carbonate tablets (2000 milligrams calcium)

Mix flour, cornmeal, milk powder, and baking powder. Cut in margarine. Mix in water (with added flavoring) and bulgur. Work dough into a one-half-inch-thick piece from which biscuits are prepared with biscuit or cookie cutter. Bake in preheated oven at 400°F for 20 minutes. Turn heat off and allow biscuits to dry for two hours. Store in refrigerator or freezer. Recipe contains 1634 kilocalories, 53.2 grams protein, and 56 grams fat. Recipe can make 32 biscuits containing 50 kilocalories, 1.7 grams protein, and 1 gram fat each.

Diet

; *ground turkey (raw weight), cooked*

½ egg, large, hard-boiled

1 teaspoon vegetable (canola) oil

⅛ teaspoon salt substitute—potassium chloride

3 bonemeal tablets (10-grain or equivalent)

1 multiple vitamin-mineral tablet

Provides 372 kilocalories, 34.1 grams protein, 25.5 grams fat
See Table 4.4 in Chapter 4 for a cat's or kitten's caloric
needs.

Chicken Diet

½ pound boneless chicken breast (raw weight), cooked

½ egg, large, hard-boiled

½ ounce clams, chopped in juice

4 teaspoons vegetable (canola) oil

⅛ teaspoon salt substitute—potassium chloride

3 bonemeal tablets (10-grain or equivalent)

1 multiple vitamin-mineral tablet

Provides 471 kilocalories, 53.1 grams protein, 27.4 grams fat
See Table 4.4 in Chapter 4 for a cat's or kitten's caloric
needs.

Chicken and Rice Diet

⅓ pound boneless chicken breast (raw weight), cooked

1 egg, large, hard-boiled

½ ounce clams, chopped in juice

⅓ cup rice, long-grain, cooked

4 teaspoons vegetable (canola) oil

⅛ teaspoon salt substitute—potassium chloride

4 bonemeal tablets (10-grain or equivalent)

1 multiple vitamin-mineral tablet

Provides 503 kilocalories, 43.4 grams protein, 28.6 grams fat
See Table 4.4 in Chapter 4 for a cat's or kitten's caloric
needs.

Beef Diet

½ pound lean ground beef (raw weight), cooked

½ egg, large, hard-boiled

½ ounce clams, chopped in juice

4 bonemeal tablets (10-grain or equivalent)

1 multiple vitamin-mineral tablet

Provides 447 kilocalories, 46.2 grams protein, 27.5 grams fat
See Table 4.4 in Chapter 4 for a cat's or kitten's caloric
needs.

Beef and Rice Diet

1/3 pound lean ground beef (raw weight), cooked

1/2 egg, large, hard-boiled

1/2 ounce clams, chopped in juice

1/3 cup rice, long-grain, cooked

1 teaspoon vegetable (canola) oil

1/8 teaspoon salt substitute—potassium chloride

3 bonemeal tablets (10-grain or equivalent)

1 multiple vitamin-mineral tablet

Provides 433 kilocalories, 34.8 grams protein, 24.7 grams fat
See Table 4.4 in Chapter 4 for a cat's or kitten's caloric needs.

Lamb Diet

1/2 pound lean ground lamb (raw weight), cooked

1/4 ounce clams, chopped in juice ·

4 bonemeal tablets (10-grain or equivalent)

1 multiple vitamin-mineral tablet

Provides 457 kilocalories, 41.2 grams protein, 31.6 grams fat
See Table 4.4 in Chapter 4 for a cat's or kitten's caloric needs.

Lamb and Rice Diet

½ *pound lean ground lamb (raw weight), cooked*

½ *egg, large, hard-boiled*

½ *ounce clams, chopped in juice*

⅓ *cup rice, long-grain, cooked*

4 *bonemeal tablets (10-grain or equivalent)*

1 *multiple vitamin-mineral tablet*

Provides 573 kilocalories, 47.1 grams protein, 34.2 grams fat
See Table 4.4 in Chapter 4 for a cat's or kitten's caloric needs.

Tuna Diet

4 *ounces tuna, canned in water, without added salt*

1 *egg, large, hard-boiled*

1 *tablespoon vegetable (canola) oil*

2 *bonemeal tablets (10-grain or equivalent)*

1 *multiple vitamin-mineral tablet*

Provides 326 kilocalories, 33.3 grams protein, 21.5 grams fat
See Table 4.4 in Chapter 4 for a cat's or kitten's caloric needs.

Tuna and Rice Diet

4 ounces tuna, canned in water, without added salt

1 egg, large, hard-boiled

½ ounce clams, chopped in juice

⅓ cup rice, long-grain, cooked

1 tablespoon vegetable (canola) oil

3 bonemeal tablets (10-grain or equivalent)

1 multiple vitamin-mineral tablet

Provides 415 kilocalories, 38.3 grams protein, 22 grams fat
See Table 4.4 in Chapter 4 for a cat's or kitten's caloric needs.

Sardine Diet

4½ ounces sardines, canned, tomato sauce

½ egg, large, hard-boiled

1 calcium carbonate tablet (400 milligrams calcium)

1 multiple vitamin-mineral tablet

Provides 266 kilocalories, 23.8 grams protein, 18.3 grams fat
See Table 4.4 in Chapter 4 for a cat's or kitten's caloric needs.

Sardine and Rice Diet

6 ounces sardines, canned, tomato sauce

1 egg, large, hard-boiled

⅓ cup rice, long-grain, cooked

1 calcium carbonate tablet (400 milligrams calcium)

1 multiple vitamin-mineral tablet

Provides 447 kilocalories, 35.2 grams protein, 26.1 grams fat
See Table 4.4 in Chapter 4 for a cat's or kitten's caloric needs.

Salmon Diet

5 ounces salmon, canned with bone

½ egg, large, hard-boiled

1 calcium carbonate tablet (oyster shell, 500 milligrams calcium)

1 multiple vitamin-mineral tablet

Provides 259 kilocalories, 32.9 grams protein, 14 grams fat
See Table 4.4 in Chapter 4 for a cat's or kitten's caloric needs.

Salmon and Rice Diet

5 ounces salmon, canned with bone

½ egg, large, hard-boiled

⅓ cup rice, long-grain, cooked

1 teaspoon vegetable (canola) oil

1 calcium carbonate tablet (400 milligrams calcium)

1 multiple vitamin-mineral tablet

Provides 371 kilocalories, 34.2 grams protein, 19 grams fat

See Table 4.4 in Chapter 4 for a cat's or kitten's caloric needs.

Vegetarian Diets for Cats

Cats have always been carnivores. They have some unique nutritional needs that a strictly vegetarian diet cannot satisfy. Cats have a need for arachidonic acid, which plants do not make. Thus, an animal source of this nutrient must be given. Cats also have a unique need for taurine because they cannot make it from other nutrients. Foods supplied from plant material contain no taurine. It must be supplied from a source where it is manufactured. In the following diets it is necessary to obtain taurine from a health food supplier and to add it to the cat's diet. Because vitamin B_{12} is not produced by any plant sources of food, it must be added to the diet. If a cat is fed a vegetarian diet appropriate for human beings, it is likely that signs of a nutrient deficiency will eventually develop.

Tofu Diet

½ cup tofu, raw firm

¼ yolk of egg, large, hard-boiled

½ calcium carbonate tablet (200 milligrams calcium)

1 multiple vitamin-mineral tablet

35 milligrams taurine

Provides 198 kilocalories, 20.6 grams protein, 12.3 grams fat
See Table 4.4 in Chapter 4 for a cat's or kitten's caloric needs.

Tofu and Rice Diet

1 cup tofu, raw firm

½ yolk of egg, large, hard-boiled

⅓ cup rice, long-grain, cooked

2 teaspoons vegetable (canola) oil

2 bonemeal tablets (10-grain or equivalent)

1 multiple vitamin-mineral tablet

70 milligrams taurine

Provides 407 kilocalories, 30.6 grams protein, 22 grams fat
See Table 4.4 in Chapter 4 for a cat's or kitten's caloric needs.

Behavioral Problems

Behavioral problems can be associated with diet. Coprophagy is a relatively common problem in dogs fed commercial pet foods, especially dry foods. It is rare in animals fed owner-prepared diets or consuming food caught while hunting. Coprophagy is associated with feeding high-carbohydrate diets, especially in German shepherds. Coprophagy ceases in working dogs fed horse meat instead of dry dog food, if caloric intake remains unchanged. Enough horse meat is fed to reduce the diet's carbohydrate content from about 40 percent to about 25 percent. The problem is managed by feeding owner-prepared diets containing sufficient amounts of protein and relatively small amounts of carbohydrate.

Instead of correcting the nutritional problem causing coprophagy, owners often feed pets something to give feces an offensive odor and taste. Chemicals for parasite control are sometimes given orally to discourage coprophagy. Sodium glutamate mixed with a purified edible vegetable protein fraction is marketed with claims for curbing coprophagy. It makes the odor and taste of feces offensive. If a pet eats fecal material of other animals, these preparations have no value.

Feeding Geriatric Pets[1-4]

■ Factors Ensuring a Long and Happy Life

Pet dogs and cats live considerably longer today than in the past. Better care, especially medical care, is assumed to increase their life expectancy. Life expectancy is also genetically determined. Life span is unique for each animal species and for breeds within a species. Life spans vary greatly for canine breeds. Small breeds and very large breeds of dogs do not live as long as intermediate size breeds.

Environmental factors also influence life span of dogs and cats. They include airborne toxins and toxic contaminants in food and water. Toxic substances can reduce resistance to disease and directly injure tissues. The greatest exposure to toxic substances is through what is consumed. An animal can eat literally hundreds of pounds of foodstuffs yearly. Thus, quality of the diet is important in determining long life expectancy in dogs and cats.

■ Geriatric Diets

Manufacturers design some pet foods for aged dogs. Compared with diets for younger dogs, these have reduced fat and possibly increased fiber. Fat content is less because obesity is common in aged dogs, and reducing dietary fat helps in weight reduction. Manufacturers give little consideration to improving dietary quality. Some believe that elderly animals digest and absorb a meal as well as young animals do. That conclusion is based on older animals having few changes in digestive tract morphology. But digestive function changes with aging.

■ Protein Needs of Older Pets

Older dogs require more protein than younger adult dogs. Merely increasing dietary protein does not satisfy this increased requirement. Protein quality must also be improved to make dietary protein highly digestible.

Overall dietary composition is important for optimum protein digestion and absorption. Dietary carbohydrates and fiber reduce protein digestibility by delaying its digestion. Normally, high-quality dietary protein is completely digested and absorbed in the small intestine, and little or no protein enters the colon. Delay in protein digestion can cause some protein to escape digestion and absorption.

Excess unabsorbed protein entering the colon is degraded by colonic bacteria to nonnutrient substances. These substances are absorbed and must be detoxified for excretion. Some of these substances are biogenic amines. Their colonic concentration increases with increased dietary protein. Thus, in addition to poor quality pet foods not supplying adequate protein for aged dogs, they can also contribute nonnutrient substances (some are toxic) because of poorer assimilation. High dietary fiber and poorly digested carbohydrates, such as in most cereal-based foods, aggravate this problem.

Geriatric pets should be fed proteins with high biological value and high digestibility. This minimizes protein residue entering the colon, where bacteria act on it to produce toxins. Protein requirements are satisfied by feeding 4.5 grams of digestible crude protein per kilogram metabolic body mass (4.5 grams/kilogram body weight$^{0.75}$) This level is 50 percent more than recommended for maintenance of younger adult dogs. However, commercial diets for adult maintenance often exceed this amount.

■ Caloric Needs of Older Pets

Food is consumed primarily to satisfy energy requirements. Older dogs and cats need fewer calories because they are less active than younger adults. To maintain optimal weight, older animals can decrease caloric intake to 80 percent of that needed by younger adults. Total caloric intake reductions must take into consideration that requirements for other nutrients may be unchanged or increased. As already noted, dietary protein must increase even if caloric intake remains unchanged. Needs may increase for some vitamins and trace minerals, but that is unproven. Vitamin E is most important to supplement. Aging is associated with many degenerative changes, and vitamin E helps prevent damage.

Older animals are more likely to be overweight than younger adults. This greater tendency is specific for neither sex, and neutering is not significant in promoting obesity. The number of daily feedings is not a factor. Factors that do not make a difference include living with young children (who feed the pet frequently), raiding the garbage, or living with an older or younger adult. The only significant factor associated with obesity in older animals is reduced physical activity.

■ Fat Digestion and Absorption

Fat digestibility and tolerance are not poorer in older dogs and cats, but aging can delay fat absorption. Reducing fat intake is not necessary unless a weight reduction program is planned based on low fat intake. Older animals require essential fatty acids, which should be given to them.

■ Carbohydrate Digestion and Absorption

Dietary carbohydrates are selected to increase digestibility for both starch and protein. Rice is the most completely digested carbohydrate. Dogs and cats poorly digest and absorb other grain cereals, the basis of most commercial pet foods. Although carbohydrate assimilation appears to be normal in older animals, in some dogs and cats it is associated with abnormal glucose regulation and signs of diabetes mellitus.

Nutrients Protecting Aging Animals[5,6]

Chemicals and nutrients play a role in development of and protection against disease. Cancer is one disease where some forms develop in humans consuming certain diets. Such a dietary effect is evident in humans eating a typical Japanese diet that is associated with a high incidence of stomach cancer and low incidence of colon cancer. In contrast, the typical high-fat American diet results in the opposite. The reason for these differences is unknown.

Diet composition can affect mammary tumors. Diets low in methionine protect against tumor appearance and growth. Foods rich in methionine promote tumor appearance and growth.[7]

Chemicals in some diets are toxic and over time can cause diseases such as cancer. High dietary nitrosamine, for example, causes acute hepatic necrosis, and chronic ingestion of lower amounts causes hepatic cancer. Some microorganisms produce dietary chemicals, such as aflatoxin produced by a fungus, that cause hepatic necrosis.

Normal dietary constituents can be toxic, and naturally occurring protectants minimize or prevent damage. Antioxidants protect against free radicals, which appear as oxygen is used to produce energy. Antioxidants are important as dietary unsaturated fatty acids increase. These protectants include naturally occurring nutrients such as vitamin A, vitamin C, and vitamin E. In addition, commercially prepared foods contain synthetic antioxidants such as butylated hydroxytoluene, butylated hydroxyanisole, and ethoxyquin.

Vitamin E is essential for cell membrane protection against the many chemical reactions generating free radicals. Vitamin E is more potent than synthetic antioxidants because it binds cell membranes. To be as effective, synthetic antioxidants must be given continuously and in large amounts compared with vitamin E. Membrane-bound vitamin E loses its antioxidant activity on neutralizing free radicals, but other antioxidants such as vitamin C can restore membrane vitamin E antioxidant activity.

Vitamin E appears to lengthen life span. When animals are given vitamin E from a young age, the onset slows for some age-related problems such as cataracts, cancer, cardiovascular disease, and decreased immune function.

High blood vitamin E levels may lower the risk of some cancers. This effect can be due to vitamin E blocking the formation of carcinogens (such as nitrosamines from nitrates in the diet), inhibiting carcinogens from reaching cells, suppressing the effects of cancer, and stimulating the immune system.

■ Phytochemicals as Protectants

Phytochemicals are the source of nearly all phenolics found in animals. The important phytochemicals are phenolics. Phenolics essential for animals, such as tyrosine, come either directly from plants or are modified from essential plant precursors.

Phenolic phytochemicals are grouped into flavonoids (such as anthocyanins, genistein, and daidzein), tannins, lignins, and simple phenols such as the benzoic and cinnamic acids. These chemicals protect plants and have beneficial effects in animals. They protect animal cells by chelating, or quenching free radicals, which provides antioxidant activity. Phytochemicals are found in fruits, vegetables, grains, and legumes; a human consumes about 25 to 35 milligrams daily.

Soybean products are rich in flavonoids. Other beans are also rich in phytochemicals. In addition, naturally blue, purple, red, orange, and yellow foods are abundant in flavonoids. The benefits of flavonoids can be lost with food processing. Phytochemicals' benefits can be enhanced by feeding substances that reduce intestinal absorption of toxins; such substances include soluble fiber.

Flavonoids help control cancer growth. The flavonoid genistein prevents malignant angiogenesis, blood vessel development that promotes cancer growth. Genistein also promotes leukemia cell differentiation so cells revert to back to normal.

Some phytochemicals are toxic to intestinal bacteria. Reducing this bacterial population decreases toxin formation and absorption.

Phytochemicals are beneficial only from dietary levels in naturally occurring foods. Excess phytochemicals can be toxic. Phenol-based compounds can be toxic; metabolism of any phenolic chemical releases phenol that is toxic.

Owner-prepared diets should be formulated with a natural source of phytochemicals. Their beneficial effects for detoxification and protection will be lifelong.

■ Feeding to Reduce Cancer

The incidence of tumors is lower for animals fed soy protein diets.[7] Several soy protein constituents can inhibit tumor growth. They include isoflavones, phytosterols, protease inhibitors, inositol hexaphosphate, and saponins. Soy proteins are also deficient in methionine. Dietary soy protein instead of animal protein is associated with a lower incidence of breast and colon cancer in humans. No long-term studies have been done in dogs and cats, but the probability is great that feeding soy protein could have the same effects. A number of forms of soy protein are available. Many diets in this book are based on using one form, tofu, as the primary source of protein.

■ Feeding to Prevent Cancer Cachexia[5,8]

Weight loss and cachexia are significant complications of cancer. Cancer patients that maintain normal weight live longer and have fewer complications during treatment with chemotherapy, radiotherapy, and surgery. Tumor cells uncouple metabolism, which accelerates wasting and poor use of nutrients. Metabolic abnormalities affect use of carbohydrates, proteins, and fats, resulting in many defects in nutrient usage.

Cancer patients are invariably anorectic and have a basal energy requirement that is twice normal, requiring food intake to be greatly increased. High-caloric-density diets are fed to increase energy intake. Up to 50 percent of nonprotein calories should be fat. High-carbohydrate diets should not be fed. To improve anorexia, palatability should be enhanced by using animal fat such as chicken fat, adding seasonings such as garlic powder, and feeding food warm. No commercial pet foods meet dietary requirements for cancer patients.

Diets for Geriatric Dogs

The following diets for geriatric dogs contain the highest-quality protein and the most easily digested form of starch. Some are high in fat for underweight animals that have problems maintaining normal weight. Others are low in fat when obesity is a problem that must be managed. All these diets can be supplemented with vegetables listed in Table 5.1. If a pet tolerates other vegetables or fruits, ones can be fed that provide natural chemicals that protect against tissue injury and aging. The diets are relatively low in vitamin and mineral content. Their requirements are met, but excesses are avoided because that can be an important cause of tissue injury in older animals. Vitamin E can be supplemented for further protection. For each recipe, feeding recommendations are based on the diet providing 80 percent of the caloric requirements of a younger dog of the given weight.

Tofu and Rice Diet (High-fat)

1 cup tofu, raw firm

2 cups rice, long-grain, cooked

1/4 teaspoon salt substitute—potassium chloride

1/10 teaspoon table salt

4 bonemeal tablets (10-grain or equivalent)

1 multiple vitamin-mineral tablet

1 vitamin E (400 IU)

(vitamin B$_{12}$ once a week)

Provides 777 kilocalories, 48.3 grams protein, 22.9 grams fat
Supports caloric needs of a 34-pound dog

Cottage Cheese and Rice Diet (Low-fat)

1 cup cottage cheese, 1 percent fat

2 cups rice, long-grain, cooked

1/4 teaspoon salt substitute—potassium chloride

4 bonemeal tablets (10-grain or equivalent)

1 multiple vitamin-mineral tablet

1 vitamin E (400 IU)

(vitamin B$_{12}$ once a week)

Provides 575 kilocalories, 36.5 grams protein, 3.2 grams fat
Supports caloric needs of a 23-pound dog

Diets containing cottage cheese are much higher in sodium; water consumption will be greater on these diets than on others. Avoid feeding this diet to dogs suffering from sodium retention.

Cottage Cheese and Rice Diet (High-fat)

1 cup cottage cheese, 1 percent fat

2 cups rice, long-grain, cooked

1 tablespoon chicken fat

¼ teaspoon salt substitute—potassium chloride

4 bonemeal tablets (10-grain or equivalent)

1 multiple vitamin-mineral tablet

1 vitamin E (400 IU)

(vitamin B$_{12}$ once a week)

Provides 689 kilocalories, 36.5 grams protein, 16 grams fat
Supports caloric needs of a 29-pound dog
Diets containing cottage cheese are much higher in sodium; water consumption will be greater on these diets than on others. Avoid feeding this diet to dogs suffering from sodium retention.

Egg Whites and Rice Diet (Low-fat)

Egg whites from 4 eggs, large, hard-boiled

1 egg, large, hard-boiled

2 cups rice, long-grain, cooked

¼ teaspoon salt substitute—potassium chloride

¹/₁₀ teaspoon table salt

4 bonemeal tablets (10-grain or equivalent)

1 multiple vitamin-mineral tablet

1 vitamin E (400 IU)

(vitamin B$_{12}$ once a week)

Provides 554 kilocalories, 28.4 grams protein, 6.2 grams fat
Supports caloric needs of a 21- to 22-pound dog

Eggs and Rice Diet (High-fat)

4 eggs, large, hard-boiled

2 cups rice, long-grain, cooked

¼ teaspoon salt substitute—potassium chloride

¹/₁₀ teaspoon table salt

4 bonemeal tablets (10-grain or equivalent)

1 multiple vitamin-mineral tablet

1 vitamin E (400 IU)

(vitamin B$_{12}$ once a week)

Provides 722 kilocalories, 33.7 grams protein, 22.1 grams fat
Supports caloric needs of a 31-pound dog

Poultry Meat and Rice Diet (Low-fat)

⅓ pound poultry meat (raw weight), cooked

2 cups rice, long-grain, cooked

¼ teaspoon salt substitute—potassium chloride

¹/₁₀ teaspoon table salt

4 bonemeal tablets (10-grain or equivalent)

1 multiple vitamin-mineral tablet

1 vitamin E (400 IU)

(vitamin B$_{12}$ once a week)

Provides 575 kilocalories, 40 grams protein, 4.18 grams fat
Supports caloric needs of a 22- to 23-pound dog

Poultry Meat and Rice Diet (Normal fat)

⅓ pound poultry meat (raw weight), cooked

1 egg, large, hard-boiled

2 cups rice, long-grain, cooked

¼ teaspoon salt substitute—potassium chloride

¹⁄₁₀ teaspoon table salt

4 bonemeal tablets (10-grain or equivalent)

1 multiple vitamin-mineral tablet

1 vitamin E (400 IU)

(vitamin B_{12} once a week)

Provides 653 kilocalories, 46.3 grams protein, 9.48 grams fat
Supports caloric needs of a 27-pound dog

Poultry Meat and Rice Diet (High-fat)

⅓ pound poultry meat (raw weight), cooked

2 cups rice, long-grain, cooked

1 tablespoon chicken fat

¼ teaspoon salt substitute—potassium chloride

¹⁄₁₀ teaspoon table salt

4 bonemeal tablets (10-grain or equivalent)

1 multiple vitamin-mineral tablet

1 vitamin E (400 IU)

(vitamin B_{12} once a week)

Provides 691 kilocalories, 40 grams protein, 17 grams fat
Supports caloric needs of a 29-pound dog

Diets for Geriatric Cats

Diets in this chapter for growing and adult cats are already high in protein and quality of ingredients so they can be fed to geriatric cats. Such cats usually prefer the diets containing little or no carbohydrate. Most older cats will not eat other foods added to their diet.

References

1. Burger, Ivan H. 1993. A basic guide to nutrient requirements. In *The Waltham Book of Companion Animal Nutrition,* edited by I.H. Burger, 5–24. Oxford: Pergamon Press.

2. Earle, Kay E. and Philip M. Smith. 1993. A balanced diet for dogs and cats. In *The Waltham Book of Companion Animal Nutrition,* edited by I.H. Burger, 45–55. Oxford: Pergamon Press.

3. Legrand-Defretin, Veronique and Helen S. Munday. 1993. Feeding dogs and cats for life. In *The Waltham Book of Companion Animal Nutrition,* edited by I.H. Burger, 57–68. Oxford: Pergamon Press.

4. Armstrong, P. Jane and Elizabeth M. Lund. 1996. Changes in body composition and energy balance with aging. *Veterinary Clinical Nutrition* 3(3):83–87.

5. Hammer, Alan S. 1994. Nutrition and cancer. In *The Waltham Book of Clinical Nutrition of the Dog and Cat,* edited by J.M. Wills and K.W. Simpson, 75–85. Oxford: Pergamon Press.

6. Funk, Martha A. and David H. Baker. 1991. Effect of fiber, protein source and time of feeding on methotrexate toxicity in rats. *Journal of Nutrition* 121:1673–1683.

7. Hawrylewicz, E.J., Jose J. Zapata, and William H. Blair. 1995. Soy and experimental cancer: Animal studies. *Journal of Nutrition* 125:698S–708S.

8. Ogilvie, Gregory K. 1996. Nutrition and cancer—Are eicosanoids the answer? *Veterinary Clinical Nutrition* 3(3):78–82.

PART THREE
Food Intolerance and Allergy

CHAPTER 6
Adaptation to the Diet

Pet food nutritionists believe that, given enough time, dogs (and to some extent cats) adapt to any foodstuffs in commercial pet foods.[1] Because dogs' feeding behavior, digestive processes, and metabolism adapt easily, the pet food industry can develop many commercial dog foods. Some brands vary tremendously from others. Experts believe that changing from one type to another requires no more than a few days to adapt. Abrupt changes often cause inappetence, vomiting, diarrhea, and flatus. Short-term adaptability depends on adjusting digestion to assimilate diets with different nutrient (carbohydrate, protein, and fat) compositions. An abrupt change to a high-fat or high-carbohydrate diet, for example, usually causes digestive upset. Within a few days gastrointestinal functions adapt, and signs of indigestion disappear.

Dogs and cats do not invariably adapt to eating commercial pet foods. The requirement to adapt begins with the first feeding of commercial food. The age of a puppy or kitten decides whether the pet can adapt. If adaptation does not occur, a lifelong problem with gastrointestinal upsets begins. More commonly, animals adapt to commercial diets when they are young but then lose the adaptation later. They most often lose adaptation following acute gastrointestinal disease, due to a variety of causes; the pet loses its ability to consume and "tolerate" any previously fed commercial diets.

Adaptation to Nutrient Excess

A cat or dog usually can adapt to commercial diets containing excess nutrients. Long-term adaptability is possible for diets with relative excesses of either carbohydrates, fats, or proteins. Excesses of many vitamins cause few if any problems. However, excess vitamin A or D can cause life-threatening disturbances. Vitamin A acting with some toxins (often found in the gastrointestinal tract at very low concentrations) can damage the liver. Vitamin D excess can kill an animal by stimulating calcium absorption so hypercalcemia results. Commercial pet foods can also contain excess trace minerals iron and copper. After absorption both elements are stored in the liver, and they are not easily eliminated from the body. Accumulated iron or copper are hepatotoxic.

Nutrient Deficiency

Adaptation to commercial pet foods deficient in one or more nutrients is not possible when no other foods are fed. Vitamin and mineral deficiency will eventually cause signs of disease, which may take months or years, especially if the deficiency is marginal. To avoid deficiencies, manufacturers supplement diets with excess vitamins and minerals. Sometimes the nutritional requirement for a nutrient is an estimate. In such cases the nutrient is often added in even greater excess to minimize a possibility for deficiency.

The Critical Adaptation—Weaning[2-4]

The first and most significant adaptation to a new food begins when a puppy or kitten is weaned from nursing, as the sole source of nutrients, to eating a variety of other foods. During nursing, young animals receive milk designed to meet specific needs. The composition of maternal milk varies greatly between species. Milk from a different species substituted for its own disrupts a nursing animal's growth and normal gastrointestinal tract function. That kind of change can interfere with the neonate's ability to develop normal gastrointestinal tract function for months or years to come. It is important to appreciate all the changes occurring in the neonate during the development of normal gastrointestinal tract function.

■ **Exposure to Foreign Substances Begins**

When a puppy or kitten begins eating foods other than its mother's milk, it consumes something "foreign." The gastrointestinal tract must develop so it protects the body against anything foreign passing through. If protective mechanisms are inadequate, it is likely an adverse reaction to food will appear. An adverse reaction can be food intolerance (a reaction not involving the immune system by which an allergy or hypersensitivity develops) or a food allergy (an immunologic or hypersensitivity reaction). During its lifetime a dog or cat will consume hundreds of pounds of foreign foods to which it must adapt; without adaptation an adverse reaction to food will appear.

■ **Protection against Foreign Substances**

The normal process of adaptation begins even before the neonate begins to eat foods other than maternal milk. Shortly after birth the gastrointestinal tract encounters other foreign substances such as bacteria, viruses, and parasites. The neonate's adaptation is the development of a protective barrier, the mucosal epithelial surface of the gastrointestinal tract. This mucosal barrier protects against entry by foreign substances whether they are food, bacteria, viruses, parasites, or even the many foreign substances that are added to commercial pet foods. Timing of the protective mucosal barrier's development is critical to when a young puppy or kitten can be weaned.

Protection by Gastric Acid and Pepsin

The gastrointestinal tract's protective functions begin with gastric acid and pepsinogen secretion. Acid alters dietary proteins so that they are less likely to be antigenic and they can be readily digested by pepsin. Acid also helps kill bacteria, viruses, and some parasites entering the gastrointestinal tract. The protective function continues in the small intestine by pancreatic and intestinal digestive enzymes that degrade carbohydrates, fats, and proteins. As undigested foods they are foreign and can cause adverse reactions.

Regulation of Bacteria Populating the Gastrointestinal Tract

Very young puppies and kittens secrete little gastric acid. They readily digest and absorb maternal milk with no need for gastric acid. Acid protects against microorganisms entering the gastrointestinal tract, but that is less important in nursing neonates. After birth, bacteria soon populate the gastrointestinal tract, with the largest number in the large intestine and smaller numbers in the small intestine. A more favorable population develops when young animals consume only maternal milk. When young animals begin to eat other food (including any other milk or formula), the bacterial population changes so that potential disease-causing bacteria can now populate the gastrointestinal tract. That is an important reason why formula-fed orphans have so many more gastrointestinal tract problems than nursing puppies or kittens. Even when the neonate continues to nurse, the introduction of any new food changes the bacterial population of the gastrointestinal tract to that found in the adult animal. The change is irreversible. It is also a major change to which the puppy or kitten must adapt. If an animal is too young for making the appropriate adaptation, signs of gastrointestinal problems develop.

Digestion of Foreign Substances

The neonate requires weeks to develop its capacity for digesting carbohydrates, fats, and proteins. Because the neonate lacks mature gastrointestinal functions, intact foods are absorbed from the intestine. Intact foods, especially proteins, are foreign and stimulate allergic or hypersensitivity responses when absorbed. Nursing animals consume milk protein that is digested and absorbed more completely than most other proteins. In contrast, an animal of the same age eating a commercial pet food must digest and absorb the poorly digested proteins found in commercial foods. That combined with a not-yet-mature digestive capacity for proteins increases the likelihood for absorption of intact proteins and the subsequent development of an allergy.

Permeability of and Protection by the Mucosal Barrier

The protective mucosal surface is also a physical barrier protecting against absorption or entry of intact particles. In neonates the barrier is much more permeable to entry of such particles than in more mature animals. Very young animals eating commercial pet food absorb undigested material that can cause allergies. Diets with many new and poorly digested ingredients should not be fed until animals mature. The gastrointestinal system needs time to mature. The mucosal physical barrier needs time to develop. Development of allergies or hypersensitivities following an acute gastrointestinal disorder is described later in the chapter. Acute episodes disrupt the mucosal barrier so it becomes permeable to entry by substances in the intestine.

Intestinal Motility—Peristalsis

The protective barrier to entry by foreign substances includes normal peristaltic activity that prevents accumulation of contents in the intestine. A loss of normal peristalsis causes intestinal bacteria to increase in number. Drugs and disease impair peristalsis and cause this protective function to be lost.

Immune Barrier—Oral Tolerance[2-4]

Complex interactions within the gastrointestinal tract and elements of the immune system are essential for protecting an animal against foreign matter passing through the gut. The result of these interactions is called "oral tolerance." It is the ability of the animal to ignore the foreign matter that could stimulate an allergic response or hypersensitivity. This tolerance is essential to life. Without it animals would likely develop allergies to foreign material in the intestine. Animals are not born with oral tolerance; it develops at a young age. Tolerance can be subsequently lost with development of an allergy or hypersensitivity.

Oral tolerance is necessary because the nonimmunologic mucosal barrier is imperfect. Small but significant amounts of intact proteins and other allergy-promoting substances can penetrate the intestinal mucosa and enter the body.

Oral tolerance consists of two parts. One is an antibody made specifically against foreign matter. The antibody (IgA) is secreted onto the mucosal surface and covers it like an antiseptic paint. Antibody binds to foreign matter in the lumen, which prevents the substance's mucosal penetration. Impaired antibody production increases susceptibility for allergy.

The second component to oral tolerance consists of immune cells, lymphocytes, that specifically suppress immune responses. With an animal's tolerance to a specific substance, these lymphocytes are sensitized to suppress the ability of that substance to stimulate other parts of the immune system to cause an allergic response. These suppressor cells inhibit other lymphocytes that normally respond to a foreign substance by making antibodies or causing a hypersensitivity reaction.

To have tolerance for substances passing through the intestine, an animal needs both the ability to secrete the antibodies and the activity of suppressor cells. Oral tolerance is lost with development of a food allergy, manifested by gastrointestinal signs. If the offending food is no longer consumed, it is possible to regain oral tolerance, and the signs of the allergy will be gone. Some drugs interfere with the return of oral tolerance, however. Drugs suppressing immune system function can inhibit production of antibodies for secretion onto mucosal surfaces. Drugs can also inhibit suppressor cell function and prevent the regaining of oral tolerance. Corticosteroids are the most commonly used drugs that suppress the immune system.

Age for Development of Oral Tolerance

Animals must be able to develop oral tolerance when they are weaned and begin eating new foods. It is unknown when a puppy or kitten has the maturity to develop oral tolerance. It is estimated that it must be older than six weeks. If new foods are consumed before that age, it is likely that oral tolerance will not develop. Feeding a new food to which an animal has no oral tolerance is likely to result in an allergy to that food.

Many puppies and some kittens begin eating a variety of new foods long before they are six weeks old. When their eyes open at 10 to 14 days of age and they are able to crawl, young animals begin eating food available for adults. For many bitches and queens, food is always available, and owners begin weaning at a very young age. This protects against marked deterioration of the mother's nutritional condition. The age at which a young puppy begins eating new foods is earlier for medium size to large breed dogs. A large litter of these rapidly growing puppies will quickly drain the mother of her nutrients. In consideration of the welfare of the mother and with the goal of quickly restoring her nutrition (so the owner can breed her again soon), puppies are weaned as early as possible. For larger breed dogs this objective is realistic and justifiable. However, owners should not wean these puppies at a very young age, but at an age that is not likely to result in the puppy developing a food allergy.

Feeding Commercial Pet Foods and Food Allergies

Food allergies in dogs and cats are more common today than before 1960. Some may suggest that the inbreeding of dogs and cats has resulted in the increased prevalence of such allergies. Inbreeding has been a common practice for developing dog and cat breeds for centuries, however. Over the past 50 years, the increase in food allergy prevalence is more likely a consequence of feeding commercially prepared pet foods. Today most pet owners elect to feed commercial pet foods. They have little interest or knowledge for preparing their pets' diets. Before 1960 most people fed their pets leftovers from meals they consumed. (In Europe food allergies in dogs are common where people feed commercial pet foods. In Italy pet owners do not feed commercial pet foods, and their dogs rarely have food allergies.)

The pet food industry markets products it claims to be nutritionally complete. The industry argues that anyone feeding leftovers is likely to feed a nutritionally imbalanced diet, one that is likely to result in signs of a deficiency. The food allergies we see today are far more prevalent, troublesome, and significant than deficiencies from feeding a diet of human leftovers. Probably obesity is the greatest problem from people feeding leftovers. That is also a major problem with feeding commercial pet foods because the industry's chief objective is to provide the tastiest and most acceptable food possible. In both cases pets eat to satisfy tastes rather than to satisfy nutritional (caloric) needs.

From a Carnivore to a Grain Eater

Quality of pet food ingredients is more important to a pet's well-being than the diet's nutritional "completeness." The ingredients listed on dry food indicate cereals as the most abundant (first on the list). Cereals, the least costly ingredient, reduce production costs. Dogs and cats are not anatomically and physiologically designed to be vegetarians. Cereals are also not nutritionally adequate because they do not satisfy some essential amino acid requirements. Thus, dogs and cats are not designed to consume vegetable or cereal products as the most significant parts of their diets.

Dietary Allergy to Grains[5]

Dogs and cats are more likely to develop allergies to cereal products than to any other food. An allergy to a protein (gluten) found in wheat, barley, oats, and rye cereals is a cause of chronic diarrhea and sometimes vomiting in dogs. The allergy is gluten-induced enteropathy; in human beings the same problem is also called celiac disease. In dogs the allergy begins at the time of weaning when a puppy consumes a commercial pet food. The problem can be prevented in dogs.

Studies on the weaning of human infants report that the incidence of celiac disease is much lower with two changes in the way they are fed.[6] Fewer cases occur when breast-feeding is the only source of nutrition and continues for a long time. For example, fewer cases develop in infants nursing for six months. More cases of celiac disease occur in infants who begin eating other foods at one month of age. The second change in feeding practice that lowers the incidence of celiac disease is to feed infants gluten-free cereals. This information should be used to develop pet foods and feeding practices for dogs and cats.

Scientific studies on nonhuman primates show that chronic diarrhea in mature individuals depends on how animals are fed at a very young age.[7] Primate centers usually wean monkeys as early as possible. The protocols for weaning describe how commercial primate food should be soaked with milk and offered as the only food until the animal begins to eat it. The animal may eat a milk formula for the first two to four weeks of life, and after that a change is made to monkey food. Although it is nutritionally balanced for the primate, monkey food is a cereal-based diet that is not at all like what this animal eats in its natural state. What is the result of these colony-raised monkeys being forced to eat monkey chow at a very early age?

Primates weaned onto monkey chow at an early age have a much higher incidence of chronic diarrhea than a monkey allowed to nurse for at least three to four months.[7] The early weaning practice causes monkeys to develop diarrhea, which is their most common problem in captivity, whether in a primate colony or a zoological garden. Little is being done to prevent the problem by feeding monkeys differently.

Puppies, especially of medium size and larger breeds, almost invariably eat cereal-based dry dog food by the time they are three weeks of age. Thus, they consume gluten-containing cereals, the most common food to which dogs are allergic, at an age when they are not old enough to develop oral tolerance. When a puppy becomes allergic to glutens, the allergy remains and worsens unless gluten-containing cereals are removed from the diet. Signs of gastrointestinal upset are common when a puppy eats the cereals at a very early age. Diarrhea, vomiting, and sometimes weight loss continue as long as the cereal remains in the diet. If gluten-containing cereals are no longer fed, these signs of gastrointestinal upset disappear. Signs of the gluten allergy disappear, and they do not return months later when the animal is fed gluten-containing cereals again. The allergy to glutens is then lost; oral tolerance to glutens has been regained. Therefore, if owners delay feeding such cereals until puppies can develop oral tolerance, no signs of gastrointestinal upset will appear in the first place.

A Weaning Protocol to Prevent Allergies

When should a puppy or kitten be weaned? What kind of diet should be fed at weaning time? Six weeks of age is close to an estimated ideal time for weaning.[2,3] For other than small breed dogs and cats, that time is impractical for weaning. Effective recommendations can be made to prevent food allergies in an animal too young for developing oral tolerance. Rather than emphasizing a time for weaning, one should know how to feed a young animal during weaning. This is based on knowing the conditions that make it more difficult for oral tolerance to develop.

■ Absorption of Intact Proteins and the Development of Allergies[8]

The intestinal mucosa's physical barrier is porous in very young animals. Its porosity facilitates absorption of colostral antibodies. Antibodies are large molecules compared with nutrients crossing the intestinal mucosa. With time the mucosa becomes nonporous and prevents absorption of antibodies. Greater mucosal leakiness in very young animals permits absorption of intact food particles. Feeding commercial pet foods when the mucosa is leaky increases the chances for developing allergies and the chances for oral tolerance not developing or being lost. As described later, any disease that increases mucosal permeability in adult animals allows easier absorption of intact foods. This often causes food allergies to develop.

■ The Mother's Role in Developing Allergies[4]

Besides antibodies in colostrum moving across the mucosa and entering the body, there can be entry of intact food particles from maternal milk. These can be food particles from the bitch's or queen's diet that are absorbed undigested and enter its milk. During nursing that milk can sensitize young animals so they become allergic to the food their mother consumes.

Nursing young animals can also absorb antibodies against specific foods when mothers are allergic. If an allergy does not develop, the antibodies will at least prevent the nursing animal from developing oral tolerance against the foods. With persistence of the antibodies and, thus, without oral tolerance, young animals can develop food allergies when certain foods are consumed.

Thus, what a nursing mother eats is important in preventing allergies in its young. Feeding commercial pet foods, with their many ingredients, to animals nursing their young contributes many of the factors necessary for allergy development.

■ Vaccines' Role in Developing Allergies

Young animals with antibodies against a certain food are not able to develop oral tolerance when they begin to eat that food. As stated above, one way for a young animal to gain such antibodies is from its mother's milk. Young animals can also develop antibodies against foods from vaccinations they receive for protection against a variety of infectious diseases. Drug companies prepare vaccines from viruses and bacteria cultured in broths containing common foodstuffs. When vaccines are prepared, the broth is removed, but they are not completely clean because traces of broth remain. Beef blood plasma is one common food ingredient in vaccine broths, so inoculation with any impure vaccine stimulates antibody production against beef. Beef is a source of meat protein in pet foods. Feeding such food to animals with antibodies against beef can result in (1) an inability of the animal to develop oral tolerance for beef protein and (2) a possibility for stimulating greater antibody production with the result being a beef allergy. Thus, indiscriminate administration of vaccines at an early age, when it is really not necessary, can result in young animals subsequently becoming allergic to foods they eat.

■ Protection in Mother's Milk[2]

Puppies and kittens receive protection from their mothers as long as they continue to nurse. Children who are breast-fed are far less likely to develop inflammatory bowel diseases and diarrhea during infancy than bottle-fed infants.[9] Antibodies in mother's milk help prevent absorption of excess intact foods that could cause food allergies. This milk also contains growth factors that modulate normal development of the gastrointestinal system. Lacking exposure to growth factors can prevent or delay complete and timely development. At weaning, complete withdrawal of mother's milk makes it more difficult for young animals to develop oral tolerance.

■ Oral Tolerance to Normal Gut Bacteria

Oral tolerance enables an animal's gastrointestinal system to ignore nonfood sources of proteins and carbohydrates. Nonfood substances with the ability to cause allergies include gastrointestinal bacteria. Antibodies are produced against these bacteria and secreted over mucosal surfaces to protect against bacteria penetration. Entry of large numbers of bacteria can stimulate antibody production, so high circulating antibody levels result in allergies to bacteria. Chronic gastrointestinal disorders are, at least in part, perpetuated by a loss of tolerance for bacteria that normally live in the gastrointestinal tract. Thus, animals become allergic to those bacteria and respond with signs of diarrhea and possibly weight loss and vomiting. When does the need arise for developing tolerance against these bacteria?

■ Populating the Gut with Bacteria[10]

At birth the gastrointestinal tracts of all mammals are sterile; no bacteria or any other microorganisms are found. As neonates begin nursing, bacteria populate the tract. Bacteria numbers increase tremendously, but their population consists of harmless species. That population persists and changes only when animals begin consuming different foods, such as during weaning. The changes include population by bacteria with the potential to cause problems. These new bacteria can produce toxins that under certain conditions cause severe gastrointestinal disorders and, sometimes, death. In neonates that have the maturity to develop oral tolerance at weaning, population by these potentially pathogenic bacteria causes no problems because they live primarily in the large intestine. Changes during weaning also include increased numbers of bacteria (i.e., coliforms) that are pathogenic when their numbers increase. (These bacteria are an important source of endotoxins.) Their numbers can increase 100 to 1000 times. Young animals must be mature enough to develop oral tolerance when these bacterial changes occur.

■ Altering the Gut's Bacterial Population

Weaning-induced changes in the gastrointestinal tract's bacterial population appear also when animals are formula fed. Feeding a milk formula changes intestinal bacterial populations even when nursing continues. Formula-fed neonates have more persistent gastrointestinal tract problems than nursing animals. This is recognized by veterinary students at the Veterinary Medicine Teaching Hospital (VMTH) in Davis, California, who, in a program for raising orphan kittens, formula feed the kittens from birth. After gastrointestinal tract problems develop, they cannot be reversed by a return to nursing and stopping all formula feeding. The intestinal bacterial population does not revert to its original state with the change in feeding. When a two- to three-week-old puppy or kitten begins eating commercial pet food, the bacterial population in its gut also changes and cannot be reversed.

One of the most abundant of harmless bacteria populating the intestine of nursing animals after birth is *Lactobacillus*. It is similar to the *Lactobacillus* found in fermented forms of yogurt. Some people claim there are benefits from giving *Lactobacillus* cultures to young animals.

(People make similar claims for the culture's use in animals with gastrointestinal problems.) There is no proven benefit from giving cultures of *Lactobacillus* bacteria to animals. These bacteria populate the gastrointestinal tract quickly after birth. There is no evidence that giving additional *Lactobacillus* is of any value. Sometimes manufacturers combine its cultures with other nutrients such as vitamins and trace minerals. These nutrient combinations are not necessary for a neonate, and when given in great excess, they could cause problems. These products should not be used.

Feeding to Gain Oral Tolerance

Before the era of commercial pet foods, owners weaned puppies and kittens by feeding owner-prepared diets. They encountered few problems, even for puppies of large breeds. They began weaning young animals by feeding one new food at a time. The list of ingredients on a pet food label shows that feeding a commercial diet introduces many new foods and food additives at weaning. It is important to feed only one new food at a time. Feeding an animal one new food allows it to develop oral tolerance. If simultaneously, or shortly after that, a second or third new food is fed, the first new food fed stimulates the reticuloendothelial system to interfere with tolerance developing for the second and third foods. Thus, early feeding of a conglomerate of ingredients, such as in pet foods, results in oral tolerance developing for one but not for other ingredients. That makes it likely that allergies will develop for the other ingredients.

In the past dog owners and breeders weaned puppies by feeding specific foods that were highly digestible. Small amounts of intact or undigested food are always absorbed. Absorbed undigested foods are foreign to the digestive tract and stimulate the immune system, something that often causes food allergies. Highly digestible foods leave little if any intact food for absorption, and there is less likelihood for allergies. Feeding only small amounts of new foods helps the development of oral tolerance. Feeding large amounts of new foods prevents oral tolerance from developing. Thus, both digestibility and the amount fed determine whether oral tolerance develops for a new food.

Feeding a new food often as well as in small amounts makes it easier for oral tolerance to develop. Doing both ensures complete digestion of foods so lesser amounts of intact foods are available for absorption. Frequent feeding is probably more important than is appreciated.

For convenience, most owners allow long intervals between meals.

Small animals poorly digest cereals in commercial pet foods. The digestibility of the other ingredients in commercial pet foods is also poor. The digestibility of single foods is highest for cooked eggs, milk, meat protein, soy protein, and boiled rice. The only cereal in this group, boiled rice has a digestibility of nearly 100 percent in dogs. The digestibility of other cooked cereals such as corn, wheat, barley, and oats is poorer.

General nutrition is also important in developing oral tolerance. Feeding a poorly digested commercial pet food can result in protein deprivation. Oral tolerance is more difficult to establish in animals suffering from protein deficiency.

To ensure the development of oral tolerance, feed puppies or kittens one highly digestible nutrient at the beginning of the weaning process. When tolerance is gained for one, gradually introduce a second highly digestible food to the diet. Following this protocol, it is possible to wean the animal without inducing allergies or gastrointestinal problems. Before this present age of scientific knowledge, common sense directed human mothers to follow these steps in weaning their infants. They never thought of assaulting infants with a barrage of new foods such as are found in a commercial pet food.

With No Tolerance, Allergies Develop[11,12]

Once oral tolerance for a food fails to develop, an allergy may appear. The allergy results from antibodies produced against the food. If the offending food is no longer fed, oral tolerance for that food cannot be regained until antibodies against the food disappear. Antibodies persisting against a food prevent redevelopment of oral tolerance when the food is eaten. Several months are needed before these antibodies disappear spontaneously, and then if the food is eaten again, oral tolerance can develop. In essence, the animal can regain oral tolerance but only if it does not eat the offending food, even in small amounts, for many months.

Summary

Every kind of matter entering the gastrointestinal tract, whether it is food or something else, is foreign. The body must learn to ignore foreign matter; tolerance must develop for it. Without tolerance animals do not adapt to what they eat and food intolerance appears. Development of oral tolerance is crucial to good health. Animal care and feeding practices affect the development of oral tolerance and its persistence throughout life. Defective oral tolerance causes signs of food intolerance.

References

1. Kronfeld, David S. 1972. Commercial dog foods. In *Canine Nutrition,* edited by David S. Kronfeld. From the symposium on Canine Nutrition and Fluid Therapy at New Bolton Center, Philadelphia: University of Pennsylvania, School of Veterinary Medicine.

2. Sampson, Hugh A. 1991. Immunologic mechanisms in adverse reactions to foods. *Immunology and Allergy Clinics North America* 11(4):701–716.

3. Ferguson, Anne. 1994. Immunological functions of the gut in relation to nutritional state and mode of delivery of nutrients. *Gut* supplement 1:S10–S12.

4. Strobel, Stephan. 1992. Dietary manipulation and induction of tolerance. *Journal of Pediatrics* 121:S74–S79.

5. Guilford, W. Grant. 1996. Adverse reactions to food. In *Strombeck's Small Animal Gastroenterology,* 2d ed., edited by W. Grant Guilford, Sharon A. Center, Donald R. Strombeck, David A. Williams, and Denny J. Meyer, 436–450. Philadelphia: W.B. Saunders.

6. Logan, R.F.A., E.A. Rifkind, A. Busuttil, H.M. Gilmour, and Anne Ferguson. 1986. Prevalence and "incidence" of celiac disease in Edinburgh and the Lothian region of Scotland. *Gastroenterology* 90:334–342.

7. Elmore, David B., John H. Anderson, David W. Hird, Kathleen D. Sanders, and Nicholas W. Lerche. 1992. Diarrhea rates and risk factors for developing chronic diarrhea in infant and juvenile rhesus monkeys. *Laboratory Animal Science* 42(4):356–359.

8. Strobel, Stephan. 1991. Mechanisms of gastrointestinal immunoregulation and food induced injury to the gut. *European Journal of Clinical Nutrition* supplement 1, 45:1–9.

9. Eisen, Glenn M. and Robert S. Sandler. 1994. Update on the epidemiology of IBD. *Progress Inflammatory Bowel Disease* 15(3):1–8.

10. Benno, Yoshimi, Ken Sawada, and Tomotari Mitsuoka. 1984. The intestinal microflora of infants: Composition of fecal flora in breast-fed and bottle-fed infants. *Microbiology and Immunology* 28(9):975–986.

11. Guilford, W. Grant. 1996. Gastrointestinal immune system. In *Strombeck's Small Animal Gastroenterology,* edited by W. Grant Guilford, Sharon

A. Center, Donald R. Strombeck, David A. Williams, and Denny J. Meyer, 20–39. Philadelphia: W.B. Saunders.

12. Wills, Josephine M. and Richard E.W. Halliwell. 1994. Dietary sensitivity. In *The Waltham Book of Clinical Nutrition of the Dog and Cat*, edited by J.M. Wills and K.W. Simpson, 167–188. Oxford: Pergamon Press.

CHAPTER 7
Evaluation of Gastrointestinal Disease

Dogs' and Cats' Most Common Medical Problems

Gastrointestinal diseases are the most common internal medicine problems in dogs and cats. Skin diseases may be more frequent in warm climates where external parasites are common. Small animals will predictably have one or more episodes of gastrointestinal disease, marked by vomiting and diarrhea, sometime in their lifetime. The most common cause is consumption of different food. Often veterinarians are not consulted because owners recognize that these problems are not usually serious and are likely to disappear without treatment.

Causes of Gastrointestinal Disease[1]

■ A History Common for Gastrointestinal Diseases

The acquisition of a puppy or kitten requires careful evaluation for health and appearance. The care a pet receives the first months of life decides its health. Often that care dictates health for the rest of its life. Prospective owners should examine an animal's behavior and general condition to evaluate that care.

Animals raised under "farm" conditions are more likely to have intestinal parasites. Factory farm operations also feed puppies and kittens inexpensive poor-quality commercial foods from the time they can eat solid food. The physical condition of breeding animals is often poor after raising a litter. Puppies and kittens from these operations are often so unthrifty, underweight, flea-infested, or fearful of people that they should not be purchased. Acquiring such animals is usually the beginning of problems.

Dogs and cats reared under farm operation conditions frequently go on to suffer a lifetime of gastrointestinal problems. They often must be fed special diets indefinitely. When fed commercial pet foods, including dog biscuits, many have severe bouts of diarrhea with or without vomiting. Many of these animals are examples of what happens when pet foods are fed before animals can develop oral tolerance. This practice sets the stage for lifelong problems.

Most very young pets do not have major problems with diarrhea. They do commonly have occasional bouts of diarrhea. Some of these animals go on to develop recurring or continuous problems. How these problems are acquired by older animals is similar to how they are acquired by very young animals (see Chapter 6).

■ Chronic Dietary Allergies[2]

A pet with chronic gastrointestinal disease (and not cancer) has clinical signs of disease that usually begin with a single episode from which the animal recovers. Recurrence follows, and the relapses cycle at intervals of days to weeks. Without any effective management, clinical signs eventually become continuous. What happens during the initial episode to cause the animal to develop a recurring problem that if untreated eventually becomes continuous?

Initial Insult to the Gastrointestinal Tract

A variety of causes result in the initial episode. Changes in diet, infectious diseases, intestinal parasites, and toxins or poisons are the most common causes for initial episodes. These insults damage mucosal surfaces so that mucosal cells are lost. As a result of the mucosa's protective barrier being lost, fluid and electrolytes escape into the gastrointestinal tract and are lost in diarrhea and vomitus. More important, the damaged barrier can no longer protect against entry by intact foods. The mucosa is now permeable to entry of any intestinal contents.

Activation of Immune Responses

Except for products of completely digested food, the immune system reacts to all absorbed intestinal contents as foreign. Immune cells produce antibodies against foreign material, and an allergic response appears whenever any such material subsequently enters the gastrointestinal tract. Foreign material can also stimulate immunocytes so they react with an allergic response after any subsequent exposure. By then, both antibodies and immune cells can produce allergic responses.

Allergy Causes

An allergy can develop to almost anything consumed. The most common foods involved are cereals, especially wheat, barley, and oats, all of which contain gluten; meats; and sometimes eggs. Of these foods it is surprising that dogs and to some extent cats develop allergies to meat. It is unknown why so many dogs develop meat allergies. Some even react to the very small amounts of meat powder in pet vitamin and mineral chewable tablets. Some dogs show allergic reactions to meat powder in heartworm prevention tablets given daily or monthly. Animals do not develop allergies to any dietary fat. Fats and carbohydrates can cause diarrhea but for reasons other than allergies.

Commercial pet foods contain nonnutrient ingredients to which animals can develop allergies. For example, some dogs with chronic diarrhea are treated by feeding lamb and rice prepared by the owner. The dogs respond well and become completely normal. Some owners find it inconvenient to prepare this diet indefinitely and change to a commercially prepared lamb and rice dog food. Changing to the commercial food proves to be unacceptable for some dogs, however, because the diarrhea returns.

Allergy to Gluten in Cereals

Gluten-induced enteropathy is the best understood of all food allergies. This allergy is triggered by proteins in wheat, barley, oat, and rye cereals. Studies in people show the problem can be inherited. There is also evidence from animal studies that the problem develops during an episode of gastrointestinal disease initiated by another cause.[2,3]

Anything that increases mucosal permeability to permit absorption of intact material can cause an animal to develop gluten-induced enteropathy when gluten-containing cereals are present. Some animals have an inherited tendency for their mucosae to be more permeable to the absorption of intact substances. Most, however, have the acquired form that develops when another disease increases mucosal permeability.

The disease can be acquired without showing any clinical signs for months or years. People with gluten-induced enteropathy often have no symptoms until the disease worsens because of an insult such as surgery, diarrhea induced by infectious agents or other causes, and even antibiotics that disrupt the population of normal intestinal bacteria. Dogs may be similar in that they do not show any signs until intestinal damage worsens. Increasing dietary gluten exacerbates the mucosal damage; however, signs may not appear until more gluten is consumed. Thus, it is not unusual to have intestinal damage in an animal that does not exhibit symptoms of the disease. (Secondary signs such as borborygmus, flatulence, halitosis, etc., may be evident but are ignored by owners.)

Gluten-induced enteropathy is similar to other allergies caused by (1) bacterial overgrowth of the small intestine, (2) parasites such as *Giardia*, and (3) other food allergies. The allergies are similar because the memory for these allergies is in T-lymphocytes.

Tissue damage from gluten-induced enteropathy does not begin in mucosal cells but in small blood vessels of the lamina propria.[3] The change resembles those caused by temporary circulatory impairment of the intestine. Mucosal cells are damaged secondary to the circulatory changes, and these cells cannot heal until normal circulation returns. With severe damage the mucosa may not recover. In other cases, dietary treatment must continue for months or years before remission is seen.

Commercial pet foods contain some form of gluten, and even small amounts can prevent recovery. Dogs with chronic gastrointestinal disease should be fed gluten-free diets. With time, affected animals can lose an allergy to gluten and recover oral tolerance for this food.

■ Infection[4]

Acute or chronic diarrhea has many causes other than diet, but they are less common than dietary causes. Causes include infectious diseases such as canine distemper, feline distemper, canine parvovirus infection, chronic fungal infection, salmon poisoning, and occasionally infection caused by bacteria such as *Salmonella*, *Campylobacter*, or a form of *Clostridia*. Other bacteria such as some *Escherichia coli* may be responsible, but no studies have been done to verify that.

Most owners vaccinate dogs and cats for protection against the viral infections, making infection by these organisms unusual. The bacterial infections are uncommon and develop as a problem secondary to some more significant disease. For example, it is difficult to infect a dog or cat with *Salmonella* bacteria unless disease debilitates the animal. Causes of debilitating disease include chronic inflammatory bowel disease, very poor nutrition, intestinal parasites, distemper, or a cancer such as lymphoma.

Other bacteria such as *Campylobacter* can populate the intestines and either cause no clinical signs or diarrhea and vomiting. Thus, finding *Campylobacter* on fecal cultures may be unimportant.

Clostridia bacteria normally live in the intestines and cause no problems. Some antibiotics can disrupt the normal microflora and cause some antibiotic-resistant and toxin-producing forms of *Clostridia* to multiply. Bacterial toxin production increases and destroys intestinal mucosa cells. Normal numbers of bacteria do no harm; mucosal damage happens only with disruption of the intestine's normal environment. Some animals can be infected with other forms of *Clostridia* by consuming food or other material containing *Clostridium perfringens*.

■ Evaluation of Response to Antibiotics

Acute (and sometimes chronic) diarrhea is often treated with antibiotics. Recovery within 24 hours makes it appear that antibiotics were of benefit. Recovery is usually not dependent on antibiotics, however. Scientifically controlled studies on humans with "traveler's diarrhea," where infection is usually the cause, show that treatment including antibiotics is no more effective than treatment without antibiotics. Also, some cases of diarrhea caused by noninfectious problems, such as a deficiency of digestive enzymes, respond to treatment with antibiotics. Thus, it is not possible to blame infection as the cause of diarrhea just because the animal responds to antibiotics. Also, when allergies develop against intestinal contents, allergies can be to the content's bacteria. Then, using antibiotics to reduce bacterial numbers improves clinical signs.

■ Intestinal Parasites

Intestinal parasites are not a common cause for persistent diarrhea and vomiting. An exception is for puppies and kittens bred and raised in kennels with chronic parasitic problems. Parasites more commonly causing clinical signs include roundworms, hookworms, whipworms, giardia, and coccidia. Tapeworms are common parasites that do not cause clinical signs in dogs or cats. It is not difficult to identify intestinal parasites, and treatment is usually effective.

■ Chemicals

Ingestion of man-made chemicals, naturally occurring chemicals found in many plants, and chemicals produced by some microorganisms can cause gastrointestinal upsets. These toxicities cause only a few of the cases of diarrhea and vomiting in dogs and cats.

Signs of Adverse Reaction to Foods—Food Intolerance[2]

Vomiting and diarrhea are two of the most common clinical signs of gastrointestinal disease. Signs other than vomiting and diarrhea that signal gastrointestinal problems often follow a recurring pattern.

Many dogs and cats have occasional diarrhea, for example, once a week or once a month. Often, owners believe that the cause is food, so a different brand is fed. A change often appears to help, but later it doesn't seem to make much difference. That makes it seem that food intolerance is not responsible.

It is possible to know if a pet reacts adversely to commercial pet foods or any other food it eats. Vomiting or diarrhea within 24 hours after eating is often thought to be an adverse food reaction that could very well be an allergy. Dogs and to some extent cats may show little or no evidence of these two signs but may show other signs that are sometimes difficult to associate with the diet.

Patterns of signs such as vomiting and diarrhea can be determined from accurate and complete histories. Identifying gastrointestinal problems also requires a knowledge of secondary signs. Being able to recognize the clinical signs of food intolerance is necessary for monitoring response to management.

■ Evaluating Signs of Gastrointestinal Disease[1]

Diarrhea

Diarrhea is the most common manifestation of adverse food reactions. Diarrhea is a change in one or more characteristics of bowel movements. One change is from formed to fluid or loose feces. The second change is increased frequency of bowel movements. Many believe that these changes define all cases of diarrhea. A third less obvious change defining diarrhea is increased fecal volume, however. Increased volume due to water results in loose and watery feces. Volume increases can also be due to dietary fiber or nondigestible matter. Large-volume feces having normal water content are formed, making it appear that bowel movements are normal.

Diarrhea characterized by large-volume formed feces is a major problem in many dogs consuming commercial dog foods. These diets are high in fiber and nondigestible matter that pass through the gastrointestinal tract without being degraded and absorbed. The poor digestibility of dog food ingredients produces large-volume feces. Poor digestibility relates to pet food's high carbohydrate content (high cereal content). Carbohydrates are the major source of energy in dog foods.

Dietary fat also satisfies energy requirements. High-caloric-density dog foods with lower cereal and greater fat levels produce smaller-volume feces. Some dry foods have a fat content of 20 to 25 percent compared with 7 to 10 percent in most dry dog foods. Large breed dogs eating low-fat diets often produce unacceptably large fecal volumes. Such dogs should be fed a high-caloric-density diet.

High-carbohydrate diets can produce small fecal volumes if they contain cereals that are completely digested and absorbed. Boiled polished rice is almost 100 percent assimilated, leaving very little nondigested residue. Feeding boiled rice to dogs with diarrhea reduces fecal volume. The reduction may be so great that constipation is suspected because no bowel movements are seen for several days. This new problem is corrected by adding fiber to the diet.

Flatulence

Flatulence is a common and less obvious sign of food intolerance. Flatulent gas results partially from swallowed air that is not eructated and passes through the gastrointestinal tract. Little can be done to control that. Bacterial fermentation of nondigestibles in the colon also produces gases, such as methane, hydrogen sulfide, and carbon dioxide.

Diets high in nondigestible carbohydrates and sugars are associated with gaseousness. Beans are the best known cause of flatulence in humans. Soybeans are an important cause in dogs. Soybean meal is used in many dry dog foods. Spoiled foods and high-protein diets can produce odoriferous gases. Excessive carbohydrate entering the colon, because of digestion and absorption problems, usually results in flatulence. In dogs with no digestive and absorptive problems, flatulence continues until feeding dry dog food stops. Flatulence should disappear on feeding a highly digestible, low-fiber diet, of moderate protein content.

Examples of diets to reduce flatulence are listed in Chapter 5. They include cottage cheese and rice, tofu and rice, and poultry and rice diets.

Borborygmus

Borborygmus results from gas passing through the gastrointestinal tract, primarily the stomach or colon. Absence of any sounds is abnormal. Borborygmus is excessive gas sounds. Gas and fluid collections produce sounds when gastrointestinal problems reduce gastrointestinal motility. Where an adverse food reaction causes excess gas accumulation from either aerophagia or colonic bacterial fermentation, borborygmus can be controlled by changing to a different diet (a controlled diet for a persistent problem causing diarrhea).

Tenesmus

Tenesmus is very often suspected to be a sign of constipation; it usually is a manifestation of a problem causing diarrhea. An adverse reaction to food often causes tenesmus as the primary sign. On closer examination variable amounts of mucous and/or fresh blood are often found to coat small amounts of feces. Blood in feces is common in dogs and cats. It is not a sign of a serious problem unless the amount is great or persists. Blood in feces is rarely caused by colonic cancer in dogs and cats. Tenesmus also increases bowel movement frequency.

Abdominal Distention

Distention of the abdomen or bloating can be a sign of an adverse reaction to food. Intestinal accumulation of gas and fluid causes this distention. Gas accumulates because gastrointestinal motility is impaired; any remaining movement is unable to expel gas by eructation or flatulence. Fluid accumulates for the same reason but also because adverse food reactions stimulate intestinal fluid secretion. Occasionally postprandial abdominal distention is the only sign of an adverse food reaction.

Pain

Subtle pain or abdominal discomfort is often difficult to assess. Dogs sometimes assume a praying posture when experiencing abdominal pain. In that attitude their front legs are flat on the floor and their rear ends are raised, in appearance similar to a stretching movement. Intestinal distention by gas causes the discomfort triggering that behavior. Sometimes distention by an intestinal foreign object has the same effect.

Shivering

Unexplained shivering can be a sign of an adverse food reaction. The shivering results from discomfort produced by gastrointestinal tract spasms or distention.

Anal Pruritus

Gastrointestinal and skin problems can cause anal pruritus. Parasitic infestation by roundworms is one cause. Anal sac problems may be the most common cause. Skin disease and fleas are also causes. When none of these are problems, an adverse food reaction is considered.

Hypersalivation

Hypersalivation is usually seen before vomition. It can also occur without vomiting. When hypersalivation is not caused by oral cavity or esophageal problems, an adverse food reaction must be considered.

Weight Loss

Unexplained weight loss or inability to gain weight is frequently caused by gastrointestinal problems. Sometimes no other signs are seen. Adverse reaction to one or more foods can cause weight loss.

Signs of Atopy

A food allergy frequently causes pruritus confined to the face, head, and feet. This type, called atopy, can be caused by inhaled allergens as well as those in the diet. Atopy is difficult to resolve, and any form of management should begin by doing what is easy and inexpensive. Laboratory testing (including skin testing) is not very reliable or useful in diagnosing this problem. The most useful evaluation of atopy is by feeding a controlled hypoallergenic diet. Owners can easily prepare this kind of diet. When signs of diarrhea accompany atopy, it is usually easier to correct the diarrhea with a controlled diet than the pruritus.

■ Using Signs of Adverse Food Reaction

When diarrhea or vomiting follow feeding, it is easy to attribute it to an adverse reaction to food. When owners do not see either of these signs, other signs must be observed to identify the problem. Finding a sign such as flatulence, borborygmus, tenesmus, bloating, anal pruritus, shivering, atopy, or weight loss makes it important to confirm or eliminate an adverse food reaction as the cause. These other signs are also used to evaluate progress during treatment. If all signs disappear, the problem is solved. If diarrhea and vomiting stop but one or more of the other signs persist, improvement is noted, but the problem must still be resolved. In many cases, the diet is changed but not enough to completely control the problem. All signs must be monitored to decide if the problem is eliminated.

■ Timing of Adverse Food Reaction Signs

Signs of adverse food reactions usually appear within hours of feeding or at least by 24 hours. A relatively rapid reaction, an immediate type of hypersensitivity, is seen with allergies caused by antibodies produced against food. Examples of this allergy include hives and urticaria. Most food allergies are not this type but are due to immune cells that carry a memory of sensitivity to food. The response is a cell-mediated type of hypersensitivity. The allergic reaction with this type is delayed: signs appear up to five days after contact with the offending food.

Thus, it can be difficult to identify both an adverse food reaction and the specific food causing it. Most people cannot remember foods an animal ate several days earlier.

With delayed allergic reactions, it is difficult to identify foods that can be tolerated, even when new foods are introduced one at a time. When a controlled diet is fed and no clinical signs are seen, a single new food must be gradually introduced. The effect of this food is evaluated over a week to decide if it is tolerated.

■ Further Evaluation of Gastrointestinal Disease Signs

Unexplained signs of gastrointestinal disease can be pursued by feeding a controlled diet and closely monitoring an animal's clinical signs. Some problems persist unsolved for so long that many secondary changes develop, which makes it more difficult, and take longer, to resolve the problems. It is important to understand how an animal develops intolerance to many foods and why it may have had problems ever since it was young.

■ From a Single Acute Incident to a Recurring Problem

Most animals recover spontaneously from acute gastrointestinal upsets, with no further problems ensuing. For others, however, an acute problem marks the beginning of chronic problems. Most dogs with a continuing problem of diarrhea show on-and-off signs. Diarrhea cycles with intervals of days to weeks. At first the intervals between diarrhea are long, maybe four to six weeks. When care and feeding practices are not changed, the intervals shorten. Eventually, diarrhea is continuous.[5] After treatment, cycling patterns can still continue, but with less severity. Diagnostic tests help in the evaluation of persistent diarrhea (or vomiting), the most common of all gastrointestinal disorders.

Laboratory Evaluation of Gastrointestinal Problems[1,6]

Many diagnostic tests can be done to find the cause or better understand persisting gastrointestinal problems. However, when these problems are evaluated by laboratory tests, it is important to advise pet owners that testing is likely to show normal results. Are tests really necessary then? They can in some cases give clues to a problem's cause. Sometimes they reveal important complications of gastrointestinal problems or even other unrelated problems. Normal test results rule out many problems and allow one to make conclusions by exclusion. So if owners choose to have a complete checkup for their pets, the tests are done. Usual testing includes a complete blood count, a blood chemistry panel, a urinalysis, fecal examinations for parasites, and fecal screening tests for digestion and absorption abnormalities. Other tests may include radiographic studies, ultrasound studies, endoscopic studies, surgical gastrointestinal biopsies, testing for food allergies, and testing of gastrointestinal functions.

■ Complete Blood Count

A complete blood count offers little useful information for evaluating most dogs and cats with persistent diarrhea and/or vomiting. Occasionally gastrointestinal disease results in anemia, hypoproteinemia due to loss of excessive plasma proteins into the gut, gastrointestinal infection, and some forms of cancer. Clues for many of these problems can be found in a complete blood count. Mostly, this test reveals complications but not a cause for problems. Anemia or hypoproteinemia infrequently requires specific treatment such as whole blood or blood plasma transfusion. Abnormalities in a complete blood count are seldom the reason for treating with antibiotics.

■ Blood Chemistry Panel and Urinalysis

Blood chemistry panels are done primarily to evaluate for disease or impaired function in the liver, kidneys, pancreas, and endocrine glands. Panels are also done to identify fluid and electrolyte imbalances. Gastrointestinal defenses protect against losses of excessive fluid and electrolytes. The gastrointestinal mucosa is normally the leakiest of body surfaces through which fluids and electrolytes can be lost. Disease damages mucosal surfaces so they are leakier and extracellular fluids are lost with diarrhea and vomiting. Tests evaluating for pathology in specific organs are usually normal. Abnormalities usually seen result from complications rather than causes of gastrointestinal disease. The complications are usually resolved with successful management of the primary problem. A urinalysis rarely helps in the understanding of gastrointestinal diseases.

■ Blood Tests for Specific Feline Diseases

Tests are done on cats with chronic gastrointestinal disease to evaluate for a few specific infectious diseases. Blood tests are done to evaluate for infection by viruses causing feline leukemia, feline infectious peritonitis, and feline immunodeficiency (feline AIDS). Infection by these viruses can cause signs of chronic gastrointestinal disease. In addition, a blood test is done for hyperthyroidism—diarrhea and weight loss are important features of this disease.

■ Fecal Examinations for Parasites

Parasites can cause persistent diarrhea, with or without vomiting. Examination of fecal samples is reliable for parasite identification. Testing for parasites is always done, even when no other tests are done. Intestinal parasites that can cause diarrhea are relatively easy to eliminate, which usually results in normal feces. When found, parasites are eliminated before other testing is done.

■ Fecal Examinations for Digestive Abnormalities

Small intestinal diseases usually cause weight loss. Screening tests can help identify them, with the easiest and most reliable tests done on fecal specimens. Fecal smears are stained with Sudan III and examined microscopically for fat droplets. Fecal smears from normal animals show few if any fat droplets. Intestinal problems causing incomplete digestion and absorption cause varying numbers of fat droplets to appear. More sophisticated and costlier tests are available, but they provide little additional useful information.

■ Radiographic Studies

Radiographic studies are usually normal for dogs and cats having chronic diarrhea with or without vomiting or weight loss. However, radiographic studies can be costly and difficult to interpret. Special radiographic studies such as upper gastrointestinal or colonic studies using a contrast agent are also usually normal and often difficult to interpret.

■ Ultrasound Studies

Ultrasound offers another means to examine the gastrointestinal system, as well as the entire abdomen. Ultrasound is limited to showing thickening of the gastrointestinal wall and intraabdominal masses. Few animals with chronic gastrointestinal disease have these problems, however.

■ Endoscopic Studies

Endoscopic procedures are useful in finding the cause of disease in some dogs and cats with chronic gastrointestinal problems. Besides examination of the mucosa, biopsies are performed. The endoscopic procedure can be costly and carries a small anesthetic risk. Clients should be advised what can be expected and what warrants the procedure.

Expectations for useful information from gastrointestinal endoscopy are limited. Usually, gross appearance of the mucosa is normal. Biopsies can show one of three primary kinds of results. First, the results can appear normal, which is the most common finding. Second, the biopsy can show some form of chronic inflammation, the second most common finding. Third, the biopsy can show cancer, with lymphoma being the most common. Cancer of the gastrointestinal tract is not common in dogs and cats, however.

A diagnosis of chronic inflammation does not identify causes, so little is revealed about how the disease developed. Biopsies performed early in the disease often show normal findings, and only with progression of chronic inflammation will biopsies confirm the diagnosis. Owners of animals with chronic diarrhea are usually frustrated and bewildered when intestinal biopsies show normal tissue. Also, the diagnosis of chronic inflammation dissatisfies owners when they are told that little is known about the disease. In contrast, endoscopic biopsies may help diagnose a specific disease if cancer is found.

The interpretation of biopsy samples taken during endoscopy is usually difficult because a biopsy sample size is small. Endoscopic biopsy instruments retrieve only small amounts of tissue. For that reason the operator should obtain multiple samples, and sometimes an animal must undergo a second procedure so that more may be taken. Endoscopic biopsies are limited to identifying disease found in the stomach, beginning of the small intestine, and end of the large intestine. Very commonly, gastrointestinal disease occurs only in the unexaminable parts of the small and large intestines.

■ Surgical Gastrointestinal Biopsies

A celiotomy is necessary to obtain small and large intestinal biopsies where endoscopic equipment cannot. Surgical biopsies are larger sized and consequently more reliable in identifying intestinal lesions. Endoscopic biopsies sometimes show normal results when surgical biopsies show disease.

■ Testing for Food Allergies

Tests are available for examining animals for food allergies. Some tests measure circulating antibodies against foods. These tests are expensive, and none are reliable for making any conclusions on food allergies. Feeding test diets and then monitoring clinical signs is more reliable than any laboratory tests for dietary allergies. (Laboratory tests for food allergies include radioallergosorbent tests [RAST] tests to identify specific foods causing an allergy, blood tests to measure levels of the IgA antibody coating and protecting the mucosal surface of the intestine, and skin tests evaluating for allergies to specific foods.)

■ Testing Gastrointestinal Functions

The most useful tests for evaluating gastrointestinal disease give information on function, not on anatomic or pathologic changes, which are found by radiographs and biopsies. Information on function also tells how to best manage a problem. Few such tests are available for use on dogs and cats. One function test determines whether pancreatic secretion is adequate to digest a meal. That test, a measurement of trypsin-like-immunoreactivity (TLI), is an easily performed blood test.

Another test measures breath hydrogen to evaluate adequacy of carbohydrate digestion and absorption. Breath hydrogen results also are useful in identifying small intestinal bacterial overgrowth. There are also function tests for determining transit rate through the gastrointestinal tract.

Information from these three tests determines use of specific treatment with drugs that a veterinarian cannot reliably prescribe on the results of biopsies. No other tests are available and reliable for gaining any useful information on gastrointestinal disease in animals.

Evaluation of Normal Test Results

As already stated, results of all tests will probably be normal in a dog or cat with chronic gastrointestinal disease. With normal test results, how does one understand and explain the animal's disease? Animals with either normal test findings or inflammatory changes found in gastrointestinal biopsies make up the vast majority of the animals with gastrointestinal disease. Other than cancer, how do the common problems develop in this vast majority of animals?

Is Irritable Bowel Syndrome a Problem in Dogs?[7]

Diarrhea and vomiting caused by an adverse food reaction are often difficult to evaluate and reasonably explain. Diagnostic tests are usually normal, which can be frustrating. Dogs who defy an easy diagnosis are sometimes concluded to have irritable bowel syndrome. This problem has other names such as nervous colitis, spastic colitis, mucous colitis, or another name that implies a neurologic or behavioral disease. Some veterinarians believe that dogs have this human problem if abnormal intestinal motility causes irregular bowel habits.

■ Cause of Irritable Bowel Syndrome

The cause of irritable bowel syndrome in humans is unknown. A complete examination shows normal findings; then, by exclusion of all known diseases, the diagnosis is made. Physicians believe that a psychological problem causes the disease's alternating signs of diarrhea and constipation. For affected humans there is no effective treatment.

Medical specialists do not agree whether such a disease really exists; half do not believe it does. Do dogs have a similar problem, and if so, what can be done about it, if anything?

■ Diarrhea Worsened by Increased Physical Activity

There are logical reasons for believing that irritable bowel syndrome can afflict dogs. Typically, dogs with gastrointestinal diseases causing diarrhea can produce formed bowel movements during confinement where they receive little exercise. With exercise diarrhea returns. It is easy to conclude that exercise is the cause for the nervous colitis or irritable bowel syndrome.

Many dogs are hospitalized for evaluation and management of diarrhea. After overnight cage confinement the diarrhea disappears, with normal bowel movements seen the following morning. These dogs are often discharged without anything being done because they no longer have diarrhea. On arriving home increased activity and excitement cause diarrhea to reappear. It becomes easy to attribute the diarrhea to a nervous or psychological problem.

Another example is a dog that is relatively inactive, with normal bowel movements, until weekends, when its owner is home and physical activity increases, resulting in diarrhea. Does this dog have irritable bowel syndrome? Can it be diagnosed as having a problem that is associated with humans if medical examinations show nothing wrong?

Cage confinement or exercise restriction for dogs with diarrhea results in fewer abnormal bowel movements. They improve because physical inactivity causes food to move more slowly through their gastrointestinal tracts. The slower movement allows for more thorough assimilation of meals, with the result being optimal absorption of nutrients and water. This results in formed feces. Thus, dogs and other animals can compensate when they have gastrointestinal system problems causing diarrhea. They compensate most when they are inactive.

■ Evaluating Patients for a Recognized Disease Entity

The dog with diarrhea caused by increased physical activity does not have irritable bowel syndrome. It usually has a dietary intolerance that is not severe so that the dog can compensate during restriction of physical activity. Many dogs referred to the University of California School of Veterinary Medicine Teaching Hospital (VMTH) for further evaluation of chronic diarrhea are sent in with a provisional diagnosis of irritable bowel syndrome. Many of these dogs were treated with antidiarrheal drugs, but none with success. Most medications contained a tranquilizer and an intestinal muscle relaxant, drugs used in human medicine for the same problem (with no proven efficacy, however). When these patients are evaluated at the VMTH, a reasonable explanation is found for the problem. The explanation is never irritable bowel syndrome. Most are managed successfully with a controlled diet. These dogs invariably recover and have no need for long-term drug treatment.

■ Management of Unknown Causes for Diarrhea

There is no evidence that dogs suffer from irritable bowel syndrome. For a dog with persistent diarrhea, a better explanation can be found. There may be such an entity in people, but if there is, the symptoms of the problem in humans are different from those in dogs. Chronic gastrointestinal problems in dogs do not cause signs that alternate between diarrhea and constipation. Other signs in people include bloating and abdominal pain or discomfort. Owners do not report these signs for the dogs referred with a diagnosis of irritable bowel syndrome. Treatment with antidiarrheal drugs is ineffective in people with the problem. How could they be effective in dogs, especially when there is no comparable disease to treat?

Most of the dogs referred to the VMTH with suspected irritable bowel syndrome are successfully treated. They are fed a controlled diet containing no foods to which there is an adverse reaction. When fed controlled diets, affected dogs no longer have problems when their physical activity increases or when they are subjected to stress.

Extreme stress and exercise can cause diarrhea. Hunting dogs often work strenuously, which can cause diarrhea for probably the same reasons that marathon runners have diarrhea. No one understands why this diarrhea develops. Its pathogenesis is different from that of irritable bowel syndrome in humans.

References

1. Guilford, W. Grant. 1996. Approach to clinical problems in gastroenterology. In *Strombeck's Small Animal Gastroenterology*, 2d ed., edited by W. Grant Guilford, Sharon A. Center, Donald R. Strombeck, David A. Williams, and Denny J. Meyer, 50–76. Philadelphia: W.B. Saunders.

2. Guilford, W. Grant. 1996. Adverse reactions to food. In *Strombeck's Small*

Animal Gastroenterology, 2d ed., edited by W. Grant Guilford, Sharon A. Center, Donald R. Strombeck, David A. Williams, and Denny J. Meyer, 436–450. Philadelphia: W.B. Saunders.

3. Marsh, Michael N. 1992. Gluten, major histocompatibility complex, and the small intestine. *Gastroenterology* 102:330–354.

4. Guilford, W. Grant and Donald R. Strombeck. 1996. Gastrointestinal tract infections, parasites, and toxicoses. In *Strombeck's Small Animal Gastroenterology,* 2d ed., edited by W. Grant Guilford, Sharon A. Center, Donald R. Strombeck, David A. Williams, and Denny J. Meyer, 411–432. Philadelphia: W.B. Saunders.

5. Strombeck, Donald R. Unpublished study.

6. Williams, David A. and W. Grant Guilford. 1996. Procedures for the evaluation of pancreatic and gastrointestinal tract diseases. In *Strombeck's Small Animal Gastroenterology,* 2d ed., edited by W. Grant Guilford, Sharon A. Center, Donald R. Strombeck, David A. Williams, and Denny J. Meyer, 77–113. Philadelphia: W.B. Saunders.

7. Guilford, W. Grant. 1996. Motility disorders of the bowel. In *Strombeck's Small Animal Gastroenterology,* 2d ed., edited by W. Grant Guilford, Sharon A. Center, Donald R. Strombeck, David A. Williams, and Denny J. Meyer, 532–539. Philadelphia: W.B. Saunders.

CHAPTER 8
Diet and Gastrointestinal Disease

Feeding a Pet with Gastrointestinal Disease

How a pet is fed is the most important determinant for ensuring lasting recovery from most cases of chronic gastrointestinal disease. That is only possible with feeding a very controlled diet, a diet in which the quality and number of ingredients are optimum for recovery. Pet food manufacturers prepare many special diets to treat these problems. For some patients these diets are effective. Most animals referred to the Veterinary Medical Teaching Hospital (VMTH) of the University of California, Davis, have problems for which commercial diets do not produce remission. These represent more difficult cases and are those for which the following diets are formulated.

The Ideal Diet for Managing Gastrointestinal Disease[1]

The ideal controlled diet should contain highly digestible nutrients, be low in fat and lactose, be hypoallergenic, contain appropriate amounts of fiber for the condition being treated, contain a minimum number of ingredients, be palatable and balanced, and be one that owners can prepare. Controlled diets are usually less palatable than diets most pets eat. The greatest single reason for failure during dietary management of chronic gastrointestinal diseases is cheating on the diet; owners continue to feed some foods that their pets enjoy but shouldn't eat. This happens because many owners believe that minor dietary alterations are of little consequence to recovery.

■ Digestibility

Controlled diets should be highly digestible. High digestibility helps the gastrointestinal system to rest and reduces the potential of foods stimulating or aggravating an allergy. Rest allows recovery, which reduces absorption of intact proteins. Rest also reduces intestinal bacterial numbers and products of bacterial activity.

Highly digestible proteins reduce ammonia production in the large intestine and, by that, help in its protection. Diets needing minimum digestion stimulate secretion of fewer digestive enzymes than do other foods, and that helps protect the intestinal mucosa. Consumption of poorly digested protein causes diarrhea that can be bloody. Associated with this is population of the small intestine with pathogenic bacteria.

■ Fats

For centuries recommendations for treating diarrhea included feeding low-fat diets. Dietary fat aggravates most diarrheas. Reasons include conversion of fats to chemicals that cause diarrhea (such as ricinoleic acid, the active agent in castor oil) and to products promoting inflammation (leukotrienes). There are some instances, however, where the fat content of a controlled diet should not be kept at a minimum (when weight loss is a problem).

■ Lactose and Glutens

Controlled diets should contain little or no lactose and low amounts of other sugars because enteritis reduces mucosal disaccharidase activities. The diets should be free of glutens found in wheat, barley, oats, and rye products. Glutens can be responsible for the diarrhea in sensitized animals. Animals can also develop an allergy to glutens during a bout of diarrhea.

■ Fiber

In most cases little or no fiber is given when feeding begins. Fiber irritates mucosal surfaces and causes normal cells to slough more rapidly than do diets containing no fiber. On recovery, fiber can be fed, and some animals may need fiber to stay in remission. Colonic bacteria ferment many fibers, which can cause diarrhea when excess fiber is fed. Dietary fiber also sustains large numbers of colonic bacteria, which can cause diarrhea to persist.

Formulation of a Controlled Diet[1]

■ Selection of Ingredients—Carbohydrate Source

Boiled white rice is the ideal carbohydrate for preparing a controlled diet. More is known about the benefits of this food than for any other carbohydrate source. Most importantly, rice is digested more thoroughly than any other carbohydrate. Occasionally an animal may appear sensitive or allergic to rice, and another source is selected. A second choice can be potatoes or tapioca. Potatoes are not as completely digested as rice, and if cooking is not complete, that causes more problems. The use of potatoes has been more popular recently. At the VMTH tapioca is used when it appears that rice fails to cause recovery. Chronic diarrheas respond well to diets containing tapioca.

Gluten-containing cereals such as wheat, barley, oats, and rye are common causes of persistent diarrhea. The basis of the diarrhea is an allergy to glutens. This is a common reason that many dogs cannot eat commercial pet foods without developing vomiting or diarrhea. Gluten-containing cereals are found in most pet foods; they are found in all commercially prepared treats or biscuits. The following diets are gluten-free.

Carbohydrates can provide 80 percent of the total diet. However, this is an unusually large intake of carbohydrates. Initially animals may not completely digest and absorb large amounts until mucosal enzyme activities increase to meet the changed digestive requirements. Thus, a change to a high-carbohydrate diet results in slower recovery if digestive enzyme activities are low. Partially digested carbohydrates are not absorbed, and that worsens diarrhea. Feeding small meals frequently minimizes the problem; overfeeding invariably delays recovery.

■ Selection of Ingredients—Protein Source

Protein selected for controlled diets can be from animals or vegetables. Used most often is a single animal protein with a high biological value, such as cottage cheese, or the vegetable protein tofu. Cottage cheese is the protein of choice because more is known about its effects on animals with gastrointestinal disease. Dogs and cats are rarely allergic to milk proteins. Diarrhea developing from feeding milk is caused by lactose that is not digested adequately.

Controlled Diets for Dogs

The following recipes are used for dogs with recently acquired or chronic gastrointestinal problems causing signs of vomiting and diarrhea. The diets provide the calories needed for maintenance of small to medium size dogs (the amounts of ingredients should be increased for larger dogs). The recipes list the calories in each diet, and Table 4.1 in Chapter 4 can be used to determine how much to feed. Animals weighing twice as much do not require twice the amount of a recipe. Doubling the amount in the first recipe provides enough to feed a dog weighing about 35 pounds, not 30 to 32 pounds. If a dog is not 15 to 16 pounds, begin by determining how many calories the dog requires each day and then adjust the amount to feed accordingly. These diets provide up to twice the amount of protein a dog requires. The diets listed first for treating a gastrointestinal problem are not balanced with respect to vitamins and minerals. Balanced recipes follow.

During initial treatment for chronic gastrointestinal diseases, small meals should be fed often, up to four times a day. With recovery, frequency can decrease to once a day. Some problems require that frequent feeding continue. Dogs with signs of reflux esophagitis often can be managed with frequent feeding, and no medications are needed. This problem requires feeding one meal in the late evening. Vomiting during the early morning hours usually stops.

Cottage Cheese and Rice Diet

⅔ cup cottage cheese, 1 percent fat

2 cups rice, long-grain, cooked

2 calcium carbonate tablets (800 milligrams calcium)

¼ teaspoon salt substitute—potassium chloride

Provides 519 kilocalories, 27.1 grams protein, 2.4 grams fat
Supports caloric needs of a 14- to 15-pound dog

Rice can be cooked at mealtime or can be prepared ahead and refrigerated. One cup of dry rice is cooked in two or more cups of water. Before cooking add salts and a small amount of vegetable oil to reduce stickiness. The cooked recipe produces more than two cups of cooked rice. Measure two cups of cooked rice and add cottage cheese and calcium. If the rice has been prepared and refrigerated before feeding, the recipe can be warmed before feeding.

This diet is less palatable than a dog's usual diet. Offer no other food for three days before anything else is done. Dogs appearing healthy other than showing signs of gastrointestinal problems will begin eating this diet within one to two days. In a few cases flavoring agents can be added to make the diet acceptable. For example, the diet can be flavored with garlic powder or small amounts of bouillon, preferably chicken bouillon. These additions are not made unless the diet isn't eaten after three days.

Potassium chloride is added because animals losing body fluids from vomiting or diarrhea need potassium supplements. This is especially important if they have not been eating.

This diet fulfills most of the nutritional needs for a 16-pound adult dog. Although the diet is deficient in vitamins and some minerals, it can be fed without complete balancing for three to four weeks. This diet contains 20 percent crude protein, which is nearly twice the requirements for this size dog. Calcium is added to levels that almost meet its requirements, which isn't necessary until remission is evident. A reason for adding calcium as a carbonate is that it helps manage the diarrhea. Antacids containing aluminum and calcium, such as calcium carbonate, have a constipating effect.

Eggshells can be fed to provide calcium carbonate. Empty shells are cooked for 1–2 minutes in the microwave. The dried shells are crushed and mixed in the diet in place of the calcium carbonate tablets. One eggshell weighs about five grams and is almost entirely calcium carbonate. That provides two grams of calcium. The cooked shells will not spoil and can be refrigerated and stored. Cooking also kills bacteria such as *Salmonella* that commonly contaminate eggs.

With remission of gastrointestinal signs, the diet is balanced completely as follows:

Cottage Cheese and Rice Diet (balanced)

⅔ *cup cottage cheese, 1 percent fat*

2 cups rice, long-grain, cooked

1 teaspoon vegetable (canola) oil

¼ *teaspoon salt substitute—potassium chloride*

3 bonemeal tablets (10-grain or equivalent)

⅕ *multiple vitamin-mineral tablet (made for adult humans)*

Provides 564 kilocalories, 27.1 grams protein, 7.4 grams fat
Supports caloric needs of a 16- to 17-pound dog

When cottage cheese diets do not achieve remission, tofu (soybean protein) is used:

Tofu and Rice Diet

5¼ *ounces (150 grams) tofu, raw*

2 cups rice, long-grain, cooked

¼ *teaspoon salt substitute—potassium chloride*

⅒ *teaspoon table salt*

2 calcium carbonate tablets (800 milligrams calcium)

Provides 546 kilocalories, 25 grams protein, 6.9 grams fat
Supports caloric needs of a 16-pound dog

This diet contains more than the minimum protein required, and it is higher in fat than the low-fat cottage cheese diet. Table salt is added because, in contrast to the cottage cheese diet, this diet is low in sodium. The amount added is small.

On recovery, the diet should be balanced, so the following recipe is fed:

Tofu and Rice Diet (balanced)

5¼ ounces (150 grams) tofu, raw firm

2 cups rice, long-grain, cooked

¼ teaspoon salt substitute—potassium chloride

¹/₁₀ teaspoon table salt

3 bonemeal tablets (10-grain or equivalent)

¹/₅ multiple vitamin-mineral tablet (made for adult humans)

Provides 546 kilocalories, 25 grams protein, 6.9 grams fat
Supports caloric needs of a 16-pound dog

When it appears that the cottage cheese or tofu diet fails, this tofu and tapioca diet is the most likely one to be successful.

Tofu and Tapioca Diet

5¼ ounces (150 grams) tofu, raw firm

2 cups tapioca (125 grams dry), cooked

¼ teaspoon salt substitute—potassium chloride

¹/₁₀ teaspoon table salt

2 calcium carbonate tablets (800 milligrams calcium)

Provides 561 calories, 16.8 grams protein, 6 grams fat
Supports caloric needs of a 16- to 17-pound dog

Tofu and Tapioca Diet (balanced)

5¼ ounces (150 grams) tofu, raw firm

2 cups tapioca (125 grams dry), cooked

¼ teaspoon salt substitute—potassium chloride

¹⁄₁₀ teaspoon table salt

4 bonemeal tablets (or equivalent, 10-grain)

⅕ multiple vitamin-mineral tablet (made for adult humans)

Provides 644 calories, 23.9 grams protein, 13.1 grams fat
Supports caloric needs of a 19- to 20-pound dog

■ Supplements

Without supplementation these diets are not completely balanced for adult dogs. The cottage cheese diets are very low in fat, including the essential fatty acids. The reasons for the low-fat content are given earlier. Manifestations of a fatty acid deficiency take a long time to develop. Any deficiency is not serious. Dogs and cats do well on a low-fat diet for four to six weeks if necessary. A low-fat diet is low in the fat-soluble vitamins A, D, E, and K. The body stores these vitamins, and it takes months to deplete them. Thus, it is not urgent to begin supplementing with these vitamins.

When the diet cannot be balanced with natural foods to provide vitamin and mineral requirements, it is necessary to supplement with a vitamin-mineral preparation. Supplements prepared for humans with allergies are used (for example, multiple vitamin-mineral preparations made by Nature's Way Products, Springville, Utah). The common supplements prepared for pets contain flavoring agents, binders, and fillers. Many of these may cause diarrhea to return. Meat powder is a common additive, and it usually causes diarrhea in a dog with a meat allergy. Such additives are less likely to be used in supplements for humans. Preventives such as for heartworm disease may contain additives with a similar effect. The chemical for preventing heartworms in the preventive is not the cause of diarrhea.

The amount of a vitamin and mineral supplement to give is based on an animal's caloric intake or body weight. Supplements formulated for an adult human supply the average needs for a person weighing much more than most dogs. Thus, a vitamin-mineral tablet for a human contains too high concentrations of ingredients for most dogs. Excessive amounts of most vitamins and minerals are not harmful. Vitamin B_{12} should be given by tablet several times a month or by feeding a food such as sardines that contains abundant amounts.

Animals with chronic inflammatory bowel disease will benefit from extra supplements of vitamin E, which is proven effective in reducing inflammation and damage to cell membranes. A capsule containing 400 IU can be given daily. Excess vitamin E is not toxic.

A salt substitute provides potassium that is lost rapidly with vomiting and diarrhea. Many bodily functions are totally dependent on normal potassium stores. For example, loss of normal gastrointestinal smooth muscle function with a potassium deficiency can paralyze motility, something that by itself causes diarrhea. Potassium's addition corrects the predictable deficiency.

Many of these diets need a calcium supplement, which can be given with 1000 milligrams of calcium carbonate tablets containing 400 milligrams of calcium each. These diets also need additional phosphorus that can be added later in the form of vegetables. In some diets the calcium and phosphate are provided by bonemeal tablets. Each 10-grain tablet contains 213 milligrams calcium, 96 milligrams phosphorus, and the trace minerals normally found in bone. If another form of bonemeal is used, calculations can be made to determine how much is needed to meet a recipe's requirement.

Do any signs of deficiency ever develop in dogs fed one of the "unbalanced" diets for an extended time? None have been recognized at the VMTH. Sometimes a client does not return for a checkup and does not phone because the dog appears normal. Often this client continues to feed the diet for weeks or months without supplementing the diet with vitamins and minerals. Problems are seldom recognized in such cases.

Evaluation of the Controlled Diet

Careful observation is need to determine if a controlled diet is effective. Remission of vomiting and diarrhea does not always indicate recovery. Other signs must be monitored to verify complete recovery. They include borborygmus, flatulence, halitosis, and anal pruritus. When none of these signs is observed, recovery is complete, and plans can be made to introduce different foods.

Gradually introduce one new food; five or seven days later introduce another food. Continue observation to evaluate the effects of new foods on maintaining recovery. With time it is possible to identify many foods the pet can or cannot tolerate. Eventually, enough tolerated foods can be identified to formulate a balanced diet. The long-range goal is to formulate a diet suitable for the animal and also for the meal preparer.

Feeding Other Foods

Many pet owners will try to first balance the diet by adding fats or oils to satisfy essential fatty acid requirements. For some dogs this causes diarrhea that can be explained several ways. Vegetable oils, which are rich in unsaturated fatty acids, provide the material for producing leukotrienes and prostaglandins; leukotrienes are the most important mediators of inflammation in the gastrointestinal tract. So the addition of oil to the diet results in more agents of inflammation that can cause the diarrhea to return. Also, fats stimulate secretion of bile acids, which, with some forms of fat, can damage gastrointestinal mucosa. Caution is advised when adding fat to the diet of an animal recovering from diarrhea.

Meat is often added to the diet before any other new foods. Most believe that dogs are designed to eat meat, and it is natural to want to satisfy their hunger for meat. Unfortunately, many dogs are sensitive to meat, and its addition to the controlled diet results in diarrhea. One reason is that a dog may have lost its oral tolerance or became allergic to meat. This commonly happens during an injury to the gastrointestinal mucosa. Also, if meat is not completely digested and absorbed in the small intestine, dietary protein enters the colon, where bacteria convert it to ammonia, which is toxic. Ammonia can also act with other factors to cause or aggravate mucosal damage.

If meat is tolerated, feed one of the following diets. If little meat is tolerated, feed chicken rather than other types.

Chicken and Rice Diet

⅓ cup chicken breast, cooked

2 cups rice, long-grain, cooked

¼ teaspoon salt substitute—potassium chloride

⅒ teaspoon table salt

2 calcium carbonate tablets (800 milligrams calcium)

Provides 482 kilocalories, 22.1 grams protein, 2.3 grams fat
Supports caloric needs of a 13- to 14-pound dog

Chicken and Rice Diet (balanced)

⅓ cup chicken breast, cooked

2 cups rice, long-grain, cooked

1 tablespoon vegetable (canola) oil

¼ teaspoon salt substitute—potassium chloride

⅒ teaspoon table salt

4 bonemeal tablets (10-grain or equivalent)

⅕ multiple vitamin-mineral tablet (made for adult humans)

Provides 606 kilocalories, 22.1 grams protein, 16.3 grams fat
Supports caloric needs of a 18-pound dog

Beef (lean) and Rice Diet

2 ounces lean ground beef (16 percent fat) raw weight, cooked well

2 cups rice, long-grain, cooked

¼ teaspoon salt substitute—potassium chloride

¹⁄₁₀ teaspoon table salt

2 calcium carbonate tablets (800 milligrams calcium)

Provides 508 kilocalories, 18.8 grams protein, 6.8 grams fat
Supports caloric needs of 14- to 15-pound dog

Beef (lean) and Rice Diet (balanced)

2 ounces lean ground beef (16 percent fat) raw weight, cooked well

2 cups rice, long-grain, cooked

1 tablespoon vegetable (canola) oil

¼ teaspoon salt substitute—potassium chloride

¹⁄₁₀ teaspoon table salt

4 bonemeal tablets (10-grain or equivalent)

¹⁄₅ multiple vitamin-mineral tablet (made for adult humans)

Provides 632 kilocalories, 18.8 grams protein, 20.8 grams fat
Supports caloric needs of a 19-pound dog

Beef and Rice Diet

2 ounces regular ground beef (19 percent fat) raw weight, cooked well

2 cups rice, long-grain, cooked

¼ teaspoon salt substitute—potassium chloride

¹⁄₁₀ teaspoon table salt

2 calcium carbonate tablets (800 milligrams calcium)

Provides 517 kilocalories, 18.4 grams protein, 7.9 grams fat
Supports caloric needs of a 14- to 15-pound dog

Beef and Rice Diet (balanced)

2 ounces regular ground beef (19 percent fat) raw weight, cooked well

2 cups rice, long-grain, cooked

1 teaspoon vegetable (canola) oil

¼ teaspoon salt substitute—potassium chloride

¹⁄₁₀ teaspoon table salt

5 bonemeal tablets (10-grain or equivalent)

⅕ multiple vitamin-mineral tablet (made for adult humans)

Provides 561 kilocalories, 18.4 grams protein, 12.9 grams fat
Supports caloric needs of a 16- to 17-pound dog

Many dogs with gastrointestinal problems can eat cooked eggs. This can be tested by feeding egg whites mixed with boiled rice and calcium carbonate. If clinical signs disappear, whole eggs and additional vegetable oil can be added.

Egg Whites and Rice Diet

Egg whites from 3 eggs, large, hard-boiled

2 cups rice, long-grain, cooked

¼ teaspoon salt substitute—potassium chloride

1 calcium carbonate tablet (400 milligrams calcium)

Provides 460 kilocalories, 18.7 grams protein, 0.9 grams fat
Supports caloric needs of a 12- to 13-pound dog

With the animal's recovery whole eggs and vegetable oil can be added as follows:

Eggs and Rice Diet (balanced)

3 eggs, large, hard-boiled

2 cups rice, long-grain, cooked

¼ teaspoon salt substitute—potassium chloride

4 bonemeal tablets (10-grain or equivalent)

⅕ multiple vitamin-mineral tablet (made for adult humans)

Provides 644 kilocalories, 27.4 grams protein, 16.8 grams fat
Supports caloric needs of a 19- to 20-pound dog

Or with recovery the diet using only egg whites can be balanced as follows:

Egg Whites and Rice Diet (balanced)

Egg whites from 3 eggs, large, hard-boiled

2 cups rice, long-grain, cooked

2 teaspoons vegetable (canola) oil

¼ teaspoon salt substitute—potassium chloride

4 bonemeal tablets (10-grain or equivalent)

⅕ multiple vitamin-mineral tablet (made for adult humans)

Provides 548 kilocalories, 18.7 grams protein, 10.9 grams fat
Supports caloric needs of a 15- to 16-pound dog

Eggs can be inexpensive, which makes them a bargain for an excellent source of protein. They are a source of cholesterol for human beings, but there is no risk associated with feeding eggs to dogs. Egg protein can be the cheapest source of protein for dogs.

Potatoes are probably the most common source of starch in human diets. Dogs can eat potatoes, but they do not digest them as completely as cooked rice. If potatoes are not completely cooked, dogs digest them incompletely. That can be a cause for diarrhea in normal dogs. Potatoes are the source of carbohydrates in the following diets. Recently they have been the main source of starch in some commercial diets specially prepared for dogs with diarrhea. That was done with the idea that dogs are unlikely to have ever eaten potatoes, so they are not likely to be allergic to them.

Cottage Cheese and Potato Diet

½ cup cottage cheese, 1 percent fat

3 cups potato, boiled with skin

2 calcium carbonate tablets (800 milligrams calcium)

Provides 488 kilocalories, 22.8 grams protein, 1.6 grams fat
Supports caloric needs of a 13- to 14-pound dog

Cottage Cheese and Potato Diet (balanced)

½ cup cottage cheese, 1 percent fat

3 cups potato, boiled with skin

2 teaspoons vegetable (canola) oil

4 bonemeal tablets (10-grain or equivalent)

⅕ multiple vitamin-mineral tablet (made for adult humans)

Provides 577 kilocalories, 22.8 grams protein, 11.7 grams fat
Supports caloric needs of a 17-pound dog

These diets supply a dog's protein requirements, but they are more expensive than the diets formulated with rice. They contain less cottage cheese and therefore are also less palatable. The potato diets are very deficient in multiple vitamins. It is important to supplement potato diets with vitamins.

■ Vegetarian Diets

For some people it is important to feed dogs "natural," vegetarian diets. Such diets are not at all natural for dogs. A dog is more of a carnivore than a herbivore. To feed a dog a vegetarian diet, use the following recipes. Dogs do not digest the primary protein source, black-eyed peas, as completely as animal sources of protein. Thus, if the amount of peas is too much for any dog, it is likely that any diarrhea will not improve. If diarrhea is not the primary problem, then it may appear. The vegetarian recipes are listed without and with the inclusion of vegetable oil.

Vegetarian Diet

⅔ cup black-eyed peas, boiled

2 cups rice, long-grain, cooked

¼ teaspoon salt substitute—potassium chloride

2 calcium carbonate tablets (800 milligrams calcium)

Provides 544 kilocalories, 17.3 grams protein, 1 gram fat
Supports caloric needs of a 15- to 16-pound dog

Vegetarian Diet (balanced)

⅔ cup black-eyed peas, boiled

2 cups rice, long-grain, cooked

2 teaspoons vegetable (canola) oil

¼ teaspoon salt substitute—potassium chloride

4 bonemeal tablets (10-grain or equivalent)

⅕ multiple vitamin-mineral tablet (made for adult humans)

Provides 631 kilocalories, 17.2 grams protein, 11 grams fat
Supports caloric needs of a 19-pound dog

Occasionally a dog will have gastrointestinal problems that these diets do not relieve. In such cases a purified diet, consisting of purified nutrients, is fed. For example, instead of feeding a starch source such as rice, the diet is formulated with purified starch. Rice contains protein to which the animal might be allergic. The following recipe contains cornstarch. The purified source of protein can be from milk or soybeans.

■ **Special Diets**

Purified Diet for Gastrointestinal Disease

1 cup cottage cheese, 1 percent fat

7 tablespoons (150 grams) cornstarch

8 ounces water

⅓ teaspoon salt substitute—potassium chloride

2 calcium carbonate tablets (800 milligrams calcium)

Provides 735 kilocalories, 28.3 grams protein, 2.5 grams fat
Supports caloric needs of a 23- to 24-pound dog

Purified Diet for Gastrointestinal Disease (balanced)

1 cup cottage cheese, 1 percent fat

7 tablespoons (150 grams) cornstarch

8 ounces water

2 teaspoons vegetable (canola) oil

⅓ teaspoon salt substitute—potassium chloride

5 bonemeal tablets (10-grain or equivalent)

⅕ multiple vitamin-mineral tablet (made for adult humans)

Provides 823 kilocalories, 28.3 grams protein, 12.5 grams fat
Supports caloric needs of a 27- to 28-pound dog

Healing of the gastrointestinal mucosa requires dietary nutrients found in varying concentrations. Purines are one substance needed to form building blocks for cellular regeneration (see Chapter 9). Purine-rich foods such as sardines and anchovies can be used to support healing. Excess levels of purines can be toxic, and they should not be added to the diet for dogs with chronic kidney or chronic liver disease. Animals with either disease have problems excreting purine.

Cottage Cheese and Rice Diet (purine-enriched)

½ cup cottage cheese, 1 percent fat

2 cups rice, long-grain, cooked

1 tablespoon (20 grams) sardines, canned

¼ teaspoon salt substitute—potassium chloride

2 calcium carbonate tablets (800 milligrams calcium)

Provides 528 kilocalories, 25.8 grams protein, 4.4 grams fat
Supports caloric needs of a 15- to 16-pound dog

Cottage Cheese and Rice Diet (purine-enriched, complete)

½ cup cottage cheese, 1 percent fat

2 cups rice, long-grain, cooked

1 tablespoon (20 grams) sardines, canned

1 teaspoon vegetable (canola) oil

¼ teaspoon salt substitute—potassium chloride

3 bonemeal tablets (10-grain or equivalent)

⅕ multiple vitamin-mineral tablet (made for adult humans)

Provides 573 kilocalories, 25.8 grams protein, 9.4 grams fat
Supports caloric needs of a 17-pound dog

Polyamines are another group of dietary nutrients needed for gastrointestinal healing (see Chapter 9). The gastrointestinal system also produces polyamines both by intestinal bacteria and by mucosal enzymes. The content of polyamines is unknown for most foods, but protein products of soybeans are high in polyamines; milk products contain low levels. This may be one reason that feeding a diet containing tofu works so well in the recovery of dogs with gastrointestinal problems.

Polyamines are produced from arginine. Thus, the diet needs ample amounts of this amino acid. Bacteria in the intestinal tract and mucosal cell enzymes use arginine to make polyamines. (It is apparent that antibiotics' reduction of intestinal bacterial numbers reduces polyamine production.)

Polyamines stimulate mucosal regeneration. Without this nutrient the injured lining is unable to recover quickly.

Recipes described in this chapter contain arginine in concentrations that are mostly 8 to 12 times greater than the minimum National Research Council (NRC) requirements. Thus, the diets would support optimal healing.

Controlled Diets for Growing Dogs

Cottage Cheese and Rice Diet

1 cup cottage cheese, 1 percent fat

1 cup rice, long-grain, cooked

¼ teaspoon salt substitute—potassium chloride

2 calcium carbonate tablets (800 milligrams calcium)

Provides 574 kilocalories, 36.5 grams protein, 3.2 grams fat
Supports caloric needs of a 16-pound dog
One tablespoon (20 grams) sardines, canned, can be added and kilocalories increased by 36, proteins by 3.3 grams, and fat by 2.4 grams.

Cottage Cheese and Rice Diet (balanced)

1 cup cottage cheese, 1 percent fat

1 cup rice, long-grain, cooked

2 teaspoons vegetable (canola) oil

¼ teaspoon salt substitute—potassium chloride

1 calcium carbonate tablet (400 milligrams calcium)

2 bonemeal tablets (10-grain or equivalent)

⅕ multiple vitamin-mineral tablet (made for adult humans)

Provides 654 kilocalories, 36.5 grams protein, 12.2 grams fat
Supports caloric needs of a 20-pound dog
One tablespoon (20 grams) sardines, canned, can be added
and kilocalories increased by 36, proteins by 3.3 grams, and fat
by 2.4 grams.

Tofu and Tapioca Diet

1 cup tofu, raw firm

1 cup tapioca (62.5 grams dry measure), cooked

¼ teaspoon salt substitute—potassium chloride

⅒ teaspoon table salt

1 calcium carbonate tablet (400 milligrams calcium)

Provides 440 calories, 27.8 grams protein, 10.1 grams fat
Supports caloric needs of a 12-pound dog
One tablespoon (20 grams) sardines, canned, can be added
and kilocalories increase by 36, proteins by 3.3 grams, and fat
by 2.4 grams.

Tofu and Tapioca Diet (balanced)

1 cup tofu, raw firm

1 cup tapioca (62.5 grams dry measure), cooked

¼ teaspoon salt substitute—potassium chloride

¹⁄₁₀ teaspoon table salt

2½ bonemeal tablets (10-grain or equivalent)

⅕ multiple vitamin-mineral tablet (made for adult humans)

Provides 440 calories, 27.8 grams protein, 10.1 grams fat
Supports caloric needs of a 12-pound dog
One tablespoon (20 grams) sardines, canned, can be added
and kilocalories increased by 36, proteins by 3.3 grams, and fat
by 2.4 grams.

Chicken and Rice Diet

1 cup chicken breast, cooked

2 cups rice, long-grain, cooked

¼ teaspoon salt substitute—potassium chloride

¹⁄₁₀ teaspoon table salt

3 calcium carbonate tablets (1200 milligrams calcium)

Provides 625 kilocalories, 49.4 grams protein, 5.2 grams fat
Supports caloric needs of a 19-pound dog
One tablespoon (20 grams) sardines, canned, can be added
and kilocalories increased by 36, proteins by 3.3 grams, and fat
by 2.4 grams.

Chicken and Rice Diet (balanced)

1 cup chicken breast, cooked

2 cups rice, long-grain, cooked

1 teaspoon vegetable (canola) oil

¼ teaspoon salt substitute—potassium chloride

¹⁄₁₀ teaspoon table salt

½ calcium carbonate tablet (200 milligrams calcium)

4 bonemeal tablets (10-grain or equivalent)

⅕ multiple vitamin-mineral tablet (made for adult humans)

Provides 665 kilocalories, 49.4 grams protein, 9.7 grams fat
Supports caloric needs of a 20- to 21-pound dog
One tablespoon (20 grams) sardines, canned, can be added
and kilocalories increased by 36, proteins by 3.3 grams, and fat
by 2.4 grams.

Lamb and Rice Diet

½ pound ground lamb (raw weight), cooked

1 cup rice, long-grain, cooked

¼ teaspoon salt substitute—potassium chloride

4 calcium carbonate tablets (1600 milligrams calcium)

Provides 847 kilocalories, 42.1 grams protein, 53.6 grams fat
Supports caloric needs of a 28-pound dog
One tablespoon (20 grams) sardines, canned, can be added
and kilocalories increased by 36, proteins by 3.3 grams, and fat
by 2.4 grams.

Lamb and Rice Diet (balanced)

½ *pound ground lamb (raw weight), cooked*

1 *cup rice, long-grain, cooked*

¼ *teaspoon salt substitute—potassium chloride*

6 *bonemeal tablets (10-grain or equivalent)*

⅕ *multiple vitamin-mineral tablet (made for adult humans)*

Provides 847 kilocalories, 42.1 grams protein, 53.6 grams fat
Supports caloric needs of a 28-pound dog
One tablespoon (20 grams) sardines, canned, can be added
and kilocalories increased by 36, proteins by 3.3 grams, and fat
by 2.4 grams.

Fiber Supplementation[2]

Controlled diets for diarrhea are low in fiber. Low fiber content results
in smaller fecal volume. Fiber can be added to the diets after recovery
from diarrhea. Controlled diets can produce fecal volumes small and
dry enough to cause signs of constipation or no bowel movements for
several days.

Fiber is also added for meeting the nutritional needs of colonic
mucosa. Only small amounts of soluble fiber are required, and excess
causes diarrhea. Controlled diets provide that small amount, and supplementation is not necessary. Recovery from diarrhea is usually complete on feeding a controlled diet, and most animals remain normal
after years on diets without fiber supplementation.

Fiber such as Siblin (Parke-Davis) or Metamucil (Procter & Gamble)
can be added at a level of one to two teaspoons per recipe, providing
500 to 600 calories. The amount is adjusted to meet a pet's needs.
Amounts too small cause small fecal volume to persist, and amounts
too large result in large fecal volume.

Cereals are the richest source of fiber. Most cereal products come
from wheat, oats, or barley. These are gluten-containing foods that
should not be fed because of possible sensitivity to gluten. Rice is low
in fiber, so eventually rice diets are supplemented with fiber. Potatoes
with skin are a good source of fiber. Broccoli, cauliflower, green beans,
and turnip greens are examples of vegetables that provide good
sources of fiber. When fed, they should be introduced gradually.

Some clinicians believe that certain causes of diarrhea require fiber for recovery. Fiber supplementation may not cause recovery but may merely mask the diarrhea by causing feces to be more formed. Feces are more formed and less watery because fiber absorbs and binds water; however, the volume of feces does not decrease. This results in an apparent but not real recovery. It is like symptomatic treatment for diarrhea using a motility-modifying agent such as loperamide.

Long-Term Dietary Management for Dogs

Dogs can remain healthy for months or years when fed one of the balanced, controlled diets. Some clients have prepared and fed their dogs such diets for more than 10 years.

Controlled Diets for Cats

Cats with vomiting and diarrhea due to gastrointestinal disease are not fed the diets described for dogs. The most effective diets for dogs contain vegetable (tofu) or milk (cottage cheese) proteins. These proteins contain little or no taurine, an essential amino acid for the cat. It is essential because, in contrast to the dog, cats cannot synthesize taurine fast enough to meet their needs. Feeding taurine-deficient diets to cats causes eye problems and heart disease. Taurine-free proteins can be fed but only if they are supplemented with taurine, something that increases the burden of preparing the cat's diet.

Based on clinical experience it is known that the best diet for achieving recovery from diarrhea in a cat is based on feeding poultry meat as the protein source. Cats are seldom allergic to poultry. Meat is rich in taurine, so supplementation is unnecessary. At the VMTH of the University of California, Davis, affected cats are managed at the beginning by feeding nothing but poultry meat.

Poultry Diet for Growing or Adult Cat with Diarrhea

6 ounces ground turkey (raw weight), cooked

1 calcium carbonate tablet (400 milligrams calcium)

$1/10$ multiple vitamin-mineral tablet (made for adult humans)

Provides 284 calories, 30.1 grams protein, 17.2 grams fat
Supports caloric needs of a 9-pound cat

When the cat recovers, give two bonemeal tablets (10-grain or equivalent) instead of the calcium carbonate tablet.

The turkey or chicken diet is complete except for fat-soluble vitamins A, D, E, and K. Some water-soluble vitamins are lower than required. It is not necessary to supplement these vitamins for the first three to four weeks.

It is possible to formulate a poultry diet with a carbohydrate, if it is cooked rice. The following diet is the same as the all-poultry diet except rice provides much of the energy. The cat is a true carnivore, and so it should eat only meat. Cats digest cereal carbohydrates such as rice, however. This is similar to dogs, which now are not true carnivores. Therefore, cats should do as well when fed the rice and poultry diet as dogs, but they don't. It may be because cats can only tolerate a reduced level of dietary starch compared with dogs. Dogs can digest and absorb up to two and one-half times as much starch as can cats. Cats do not recover as well on this diet as on the all-poultry diet.

Rice and Poultry Diet for Growing or Adult Cat with Diarrhea

½ cup rice, long-grain, cooked

6 ounces ground turkey (raw weight), cooked

1½ calcium carbonate tablets (600 milligrams calcium)

⅒ multiple vitamin-mineral tablet (made for adult humans)

Provides 387 calories, 32.3 grams protein, 17.4 grams fat
Supports caloric needs of a 12-pound cat

When the cat recovers, give two and one-half bonemeal tablets (10-grain or equivalent) instead of the calcium carbonate tablet.

A whole turkey or parts of the turkey (including bones) can be cooked and ground before feeding. This provides the required minerals calcium and phosphorus in their proper amounts. In that case the bonemeal tablets should not be given.

Sometimes lamb or chicken is recommended instead of turkey. Other recipes include vegetable oil, but that is not necessary with the turkey diet. The addition of lamb baby food or small quantities of liver (one-half ounce to improve palatability) is sometimes recommended. Neither is necessary. Many feed human baby foods to sick cats. These foods are not complete for meeting a cat's nutritional needs. In addition, recent studies criticize these foods for human consumption. The studies show the foods to be loaded with fillers, extenders, and water. They also can contain onion, which causes Heinz body anemia in cats. The most important reason for not feeding baby foods is that they are not balanced diets.

Diarrhea and other gastrointestinal diseases are common in cats, and cats outnumber dogs as family pets. However, no pet food manufacturer formulates a diet for feline gastrointestinal diseases. Sometimes a pet food company recommends one of its specialty products as useful for managing diarrhea, but it is not effective for recovery, however. Most of the specialty products are canned foods, and since some cats suffer from chronic diarrhea merely because they eat dry cat foods (the reason for this is unknown), a change to any canned cat food results in recovery. Cats cannot be fed the specialty products prepared for dogs with chronic gastrointestinal disease; dog foods are deficient in protein and taurine.

Some cats must eat controlled diets indefinitely to maintain recovery from gastrointestinal problems. Then it is necessary to ensure that the diets contain all the necessary nutrients. Use the poultry diet to build on; cats have no requirement for carbohydrates and so do not need rice or any other form of carbohydrate. Low-fat ground turkey or chicken will need additional fat, added most easily as vegetable oil. Approximately one-half to one teaspoon vegetable oil is added daily. A vitamin-mineral supplement is the only other addition needed to balance the diet. A fraction of a human vitamin-mineral preparation is used. A high-potency preparation not containing vitamins A and D can be divided so the cat receives the equivalent of one-tenth of a tablet daily. To supplement vitamins A and D, give one-fifth of a complete supplement once every week or two. Deficiencies of these vitamins are rarely seen in an adult cat.

For the cat there is no known requirement for fiber.

Management to Prevent Bloat (Acute Gastric Dilation)[3]

Bloat is a common and serious problem that most often affects larger breed dogs. Its frequency is 7 to 10 percent for Great Danes and Irish setters, two breeds at high risk for developing the problem. Other high-risk breeds include the Saint Bernard, weimaraner, Gordon setter, standard poodle, basset hound, Doberman pinscher, Old English sheepdog, and many others. Bloat is a major problem because about 30 percent of affected dogs die, despite anything done. The cause of bloat is unknown. Dogs at highest risk have a body conformation that includes a deep and narrow chest. Many breeders and dog owners believe that feeding dry dog food increases the risk of bloat. Nearly all owners of larger breed dogs feed them commercial dry dog foods. What can be done to prevent bloat in a high-risk dog?

Bloat appears to have become much more common since 1950, when the feeding of dry dog foods became popular. However, no one has proven one way or another that bloat is caused by feeding dry dog food. Until more is known the recommendation should continue not to feed dry food or to feed it often in small amounts. As an alternate the dog's diet can be prepared by the owner. Any one of the diets in Chapter 5 can be fed. The higher-caloric-density diets are better because the volume of food required is less than in a low-caloric-density diet. Thus, the diet fed should be relatively high in fat and low in carbohydrates (cereals, pasta, potatoes, etc.).

Universal recommendations to prevent bloat include feeding more frequent and smaller meals per day. Most experts also recommend restricting exercise before and after meals. No drug therapy can prevent bloat.

References

1. Guilford, W. Grant. 1996. Nutritional management of gastrointestinal diseases. In *Strombeck's Small Animal Gastroenterology*, 2d ed., edited by W. Grant Guilford, Sharon A. Center, Donald R. Strombeck, David A. Williams, and Denny J. Meyer, 889–910. Philadelphia: W.B. Saunders.

2. Bauer, John E. and Ian E. Maskell. 1994. Dietary fibre: Perspectives in clinical management. In *The Waltham Book of Clinical Nutrition of the Dog and Cat*, edited by J.M. Wills and K.W. Simpson, 87–104. Oxford: Pergamon Press.

3. Glickman, Lawrence T., Nita W. Glickman, Diana Schellenberg, Cynthia Perez, William R. Widmer, Gary C. Lantz, Qi-long Yi, and Tim Emerick. 1995. Epidemiologic studies of bloat in dogs. *Veterinary Previews* 2(2):10–15.

CHAPTER 9
Digestive Tract Environment: Protection of Its Integrity

Skin and hair coat provide an important protective barrier that prevents harm to the body from sun, wind, bacteria, toxins, and other environmental insults. The gastrointestinal mucosa requires a better protective barrier. Intestinal contents include greater concentrations and varieties of toxins and bacteria than ever contact the skin. For example, colonic contents contain tremendous numbers of bacteria that are in constant contact with colonic mucosal cells. Such contamination would never be found on a pet's skin. Mucosal protection thus requires more than the simple barrier of a single layer of cells lining the entire digestive tract.

The Normal Intestinal Mucosa[1,2]

The gastrointestinal mucosa, separating and protecting against substances passing through, functions in a state of "physiological inflammation."[3] This normal state can also be described as one of perpetually controlled inflammation. A constant presence of inflammatory cells is necessary to mount any needed inflammatory response and to respond to the many foreign substances entering the body from gut contents. Examination of the mucosa from a normal animal shows inflammatory cells are always present. The question is, what degree of change represents inflammatory bowel disease? Also, what are the reasons for this tissue having the potential for an immediate inflammatory response?

Prostaglandins also protect the gastrointestinal mucosa. These hormone-like substances are the most important chemicals for maintaining mucosal integrity. Some drugs reduce prostaglandin production. They are all nonsteroidal antiinflammatory drugs for managing inflammation. Their persistent use can damage and ulcerate the gastrointestinal mucosa. The most important inflammatory mediators in the digestive tract are leukotrienes. Antiinflammatory drugs used for managing gastrointestinal mucosal inflammation do not reduce leukotriene production.

How Intestinal Mucosal Disease Develops[4]

The development of intestinal tract disease entails an interaction between changes in intestinal permeability, events and substances in the intestinal contents, and mucosal defense mechanisms.

■ Mucosal Permeability Changes

Mucosal permeability increases early with intestinal disease and causes signs of vomiting and/or diarrhea. Increased permeability eases entry for intestinal contents. Antiinflammatory drugs, such as corticosteroids, inhibit prostaglandin production and prolong permeability increases. Endotoxin produced by intestinal bacteria or contaminating commercial pet food increases mucosal permeability. Gastrointestinal problems can also be secondary to diseases such as diabetes mellitus that increase intestinal permeability.

■ Damage by Intestinal Contents

Intestinal contents that contribute to mucosal disease include bile, pancreatic enzymes, bacteria and their degradation products, and chemicals such as food additives, drugs, and ammonia. Also included are undigested foods that enter the mucosa because of increased permeability. Some drugs such as corticosteroids can alter the bacterial composition of intestinal contents as well as increase mucosal permeability. The bacterial composition changes to one where the numbers of endotoxin producers (gram negative aerobes) increase. Both these bacteria and the endotoxin they produce can damage the mucosa. The damage produced by intestinal contents and leading to inflammation of the mucosa (more than physiological—constituting disease) is an exaggerated or uncontrolled response.

Effects of Dietary Fat on Mucosal Cells

Low-fat diets are used to treat inflammatory bowel disease because fat indirectly reduces mucosal cell viability. Dietary fat potently stimulates pancreatic secretion. That secretion consists of proteolytic enzymes that can degrade mucosal cells as well as dietary proteins. The mucosal cells' life span shortens, and they turn over more rapidly.

Dietary fat also stimulates bile release, with greater amounts releasing more bile. Bile also shortens the life span of mucosal cells. High-fat diets reduce small intestinal bile reabsorption, and so more bile enters the colon. Besides directly damaging mucosal cells, colonic bacteria change bile salts to compounds with greater potential for damaging colonic mucosa. Calcium and fiber reduce colonic-free bile acid levels and are sometimes used for that purpose.

Disease Potentiated by Ammonia[5]

Production of Ammonia from Protein

Colonic disease depends on levels of protein and other nitrogenous substances in colonic contents. Colonic bacteria produce ammonia by degrading protein and urea. The potential for colonic disease increases with high ammonia levels.

Little protein enters the colon when dietary proteins are optimally digested and absorbed in the small intestine. Feeding proteins with digestibility of less than 70 percent causes diarrhea because more protein is available for ammonia formation in the colon. Also, when dietary protein is excessive, more escapes assimilation and enters the colon for conversion to ammonia.

Production of Ammonia from Urea

Urea is the excretory product of assimilated protein that exceeds the needs for building tissue. Urea is synthesized from ammonia in the liver and is excreted by the kidneys. Urea as a small molecule easily crosses cell membranes, and significant amounts enter the colon, where bacteria convert it to ammonia. The body converts about 20 percent of its total urea to ammonia each day. The amount of protein consumed determines how much urea is produced daily. Thus, a high-protein diet produces more urea and from it more ammonia in the colon.

Ammonia Damages Mucosal Cells

Ammonia adversely affects the life span of colonic mucosal cells. With ammonia present mucosal cells live less than two days. That time more than doubles when no ammonia is present. Increased blood urea concentration leading to an increased colon ammonia level magnifies the risk for colonic mucosal ulceration. Thus, reducing ammonia content is important in preventing colonic disease. It is also crucial for healing of colonic mucosa during management of colitis. Reducing ammonia in the colon can also affect survival. Radiation for cancer therapy can cause fatal colitis, but animals survive when the colonic ammonia content is low.

Colitis has many different causes. One is consumption of a product of seaweed, carrageenan, which is an additive in some commercial pet foods. Studies show that carrageenan does not produce colitis in an animal where the colonic level of ammonia is very low. It is likely that many other substances entering the colon contribute to colitis but only if ammonia is present. Consumers are generally ignorant that diets contain substances like carrageenan.

Increased colonic ammonia concentrations can increase mucosal permeability without causing any signs of colitis, at least during the onset of damage. The increased permeability allows absorption of substances that do not normally enter the body. These substances include dietary constituents and products of bacterial activity that can promote allergies and endotoxemia, respectively.

Something can be done about reducing colonic ammonia levels to prevent colitis or help recovery from it. That depends on what a dog or cat is fed.

Promoters of Inflammation in Intestinal Contents[2]

Although it is unlikely a cause can be identified for specific cases of intestinal mucosal disease, much is known about factors necessary for its development. The most common mucosal changes are inflammatory. Intestinal contents contain all the factors for inflammation developing. If the factors can be controlled, it is possible to manage or solve the problem.

Controlled diets reduce persistent mucosal inflammation because they can drastically change events and substances in intestinal contents. Controlled diets are more effective than drugs for controlling inflammation. Drugs do little to control environments around intestinal mucosa.

■ Mucosal Defense Mechanisms[6]

Bacteria in intestinal contents are essential for disease to develop. Many defense mechanisms prevent bacterial damage. Peristalsis must continuously move food through the digestive system to protect against bacterial invasion and damage. Some protection depends on the diet. All nutritional needs can be met by total parenteral nutrition, but this reduces mucosal integrity so that bacteria can invade the mucosa. Dietary constituents that prevent bacterial translocation include nonfermentable fiber and specific nutrients such as glutamine.

Glutamine is abundant in proteins. This amino acid is important for energy and increasing blood flow in the intestinal mucosa. Glutamine deficiency changes mucosal cell structure and function, causing atrophy and increasing permeability, and immunologic barriers are impaired. Glutamine also helps protect the mucosa during chemotherapy for cancer. Thus, what is fed to an animal is important when its intestinal mucosa is damaged.

Managing Intestinal Mucosal Disease

What can be done about the three factors contributing to mucosal diseases? First, mucosal permeability can decrease with management. Mucosal permeability depends on how an animal is fed. Feeding must be oral, using a diet containing highly digestible proteins. Second, remission of inflammation, which follows feeding a controlled diet, coincides with reduced mucosal permeability. Any protein and energy deficiency must be corrected to reduce bacterial translocation. Third, protein deficiency also impairs the animal's immune defenses.

The diet should contain some nonfermentable fiber (to reduce bacterial translocation) and fermentable fiber to provide for colonic nutritional needs.[7,8] The products of bacterial fermentation of fiber, short chain fatty acids, are essential for normal colonic mucosal structure and function. Without short chain fatty acids, colonic blood flow, motility, and fluid absorption are not normal, and colitis develops.

Mucosal permeability also depends on endotoxins in intestinal contents.[9] Endotoxin levels reflect aerobic bacterial numbers in the intestine. Disease often increases total numbers of intestinal bacteria and shifts the population to endotoxin-producing bacteria. Certain diets reduce numbers of these bacteria and thus their endotoxin levels. Diets can thereby improve mucosal damage caused by a disrupted bacterial population. Commercial pet foods made from unwholesome ingredients can contain preformed endotoxins and contribute to disease.

Feeding highly digestible noncereal sources of protein and correct amounts of protein is important for reducing colonic ammonia levels.

No drugs are given unless they are essential to recovery. A very potent drug, cyclosporine, which reduces inflammation and immune responses, worsens some cases of colitis.

An excess of some dietary ingredients can promote inflammation. Fish oil is one example. Any fish or vegetable oil must be supplemented with vitamin E to minimize damage from rancidity in the oil. A more complete discussion follows.

Diets for Managing Intestinal Damage

Predigested and highly digestible diets protect the mucosa from problems other than inflammatory diseases. The intestinal mucosa is susceptible to damage during chemotherapy and in burn patients. Highly digestible diets protect by increasing the life span of mucosal cells damaged by the injury. Mucosal cell structure and function recover slowly when the animal eats conventional pet foods. Feeding a controlled diet based on cottage cheese or tofu and boiled rice or tapioca provides a highly digestible diet and is beneficial. Predigested elemental diets are seldom required. They are expensive and poorly accepted because of their marginal palatability. Supplementing special diets with glutamine may hasten mucosal recovery.

Dogs with chronic diarrhea, due to an unknown cause and so probably representing a dietary allergy, respond better to eating cottage cheese- or tofu-based diets than to eating any other source of protein. The very high digestibility of cottage cheese contributes to its usefulness. The digestibility of tofu may not be as great, but tofu has some unique properties for protecting intestinal mucosa.

Certain anticancer drugs invariably cause anorexia and diarrhea because they damage intestinal mucosa. That damage occurs while feeding a controlled diet containing milk protein (cottage cheese or casein). While feeding soybean protein (such as tofu), the drug causes no damage.[10] This protein protects the intestinal mucosa. Tofu diets will be more widely fed when these beneficial effects are better known. Humans with needs for bowel rest, efficient digestion and absorption, and digestive tract disease are often fed an enteral diet. Proteins in enteral diets are almost invariably of two kinds, soybean protein, such as in tofu, and casein, which is the most important protein in milk or cottage cheese.

Management of chronic gastric disease usually includes drugs for reducing gastric acid secretion. Diets can also reduce acid secretion. Meat-based diets stimulate greater gastric acid secretion than soybean protein (tofu) diets.[11] Tofu is the best protein to feed animals with gastric disease.

Low-fat diets are usually fed to animals with inflammatory bowel disease. When the total fat content of the diet is very low, animals recover well compared with when they eat diets with 12 to 30 percent fat as the total calories. When dietary fats are mostly saturated, the response to dietary management of inflammatory bowel disease is good compared with the response to diets high in unsaturated fatty acids.[12] Feeding a high concentration of linoleic acid (such as corn oil) impairs recovery. Feeding a diet low in unsaturated fatty acids results in essential fatty acid deficiency. The consequence of the latter is less harmful than inflammatory bowel disease.

■ Fish Oil Diet for Managing Digestive Tract Disease

Special canine diets have been formulated with relatively large amounts of fish oil and marketed with the claim that they are beneficial for management of some inflammatory diseases. There are no clinical studies to show they are beneficial. In addition diets containing fish oil have a strong and offensive odor.

Fish Oil's Effects on Inflammation[13]

Small animals require unsaturated fatty acids to produce the most important mediators of inflammation (leukotrienes). Some fatty acids (omega-3) produce leukotrienes possessing a weaker ability to provoke inflammation than those made from the most abundant (omega-6) fatty acids. Fish oils have the highest concentrations of omega-3 fatty acids (with a few exceptions such as flax seed oil), which produce the less potent leukotrienes.

Some pet food producers recommend feeding high concentrations of omega-3 fatty acid–rich oils to manage inflammation. This reduces the formation of more potent leukotrienes. Theoretically, fortification with omega-3 fatty acids should aid in recovery from any type of inflammation. However, diets enriched with highly unsaturated fats such as fish oil can cause intestinal inflammation. One reason is that fish oil diets reduce mucosal concentrations of prostaglandins. Prostaglandins are cytoprotective for gastrointestinal mucosa.

The effects of reduced mucosal prostaglandin protection can be prevented by dietary antioxidants. High unsaturated fatty acid levels deplete compounds needed to protect against oxidative stress (formation of oxygen-free radicals that destroy living tissue).[14] Diets with high unsaturated fatty acid levels must contain additional antioxidants such as vitamin E. A high–fish oil diet must contain more than the usual amounts of vitamin E. Supplementation with vitamin E in animals with inflammatory bowel disease reduces mucosal damage. The beneficial effects of feeding omega-3 fatty acids may be negligible, and any improvement is probably due to vitamin E acting as an antioxidant. It is much easier and less expensive to formulate a diet with vitamin E and no fish oil.

Fish Oil–Enriched Commercial Pet Foods

Some manufacturers fortify pet foods with fish oil and recommend them for animals with skin disease such as pruritus due to fleas, allergies, and other inflammatory conditions. They also recommend these diets for management of gastrointestinal problems due to suspected food allergy and inflammatory diseases. The companies fortify the diets with omega-3 fatty acids so that the ratio of omega-6 to omega-3 fatty acids is between 5 to 1 and 10 to 1. Scientists evaluated the effects of feeding this diet by measuring concentrations of weakly and strongly proinflammatory leukotrienes in canine skin and some white blood cells.[15] They found the diet reduces the strongly and increases the weakly proinflammatory leukotriene concentrations. Do these changes improve clinical signs of skin or gastrointestinal disease?

Fish Oil Benefits Are Unproven

There are no studies evaluating clinical responses to feeding fish oil–enriched diets. They are of no proven benefit for skin or gastrointestinal diseases. Yet a pet food manufacturer promotes such products with the statement:

> *Continuing research provides compelling new insight into the effective dietary management of hypersensitivity. To help manage inflammation and pruritus in animals afflicted with common hypersensitivity disease, research strongly indicates that veterinarians and their clients should choose diets with optimal omega-6:omega-3 fatty acid ratios (5:1 to 10:1) and limited, highly digestible protein sources.*[16]

Scientists studying human problems conduct most of the research on these diets. In the review "Evolving Medical Therapies for

Inflammatory Bowel Disease," the author states:

> *Other potential sites of eicosanoid inhibition include the diversion of mediators away from the 5-LO pathway to less "pro-inflammatory" derivatives as has been accomplished to a modest degree by the administration of high concentrations of omega-3 fatty acids (fish oils). Clinical trials using high doses have demonstrated more biochemical effects than clinical benefits. The latter are overcome by a fishy odor and potential impact on coagulation.*[17]

In summary, the fish oil diets show questionable clinical benefits, are smelly, and can cause problems by promoting bleeding. Diets rich in unsaturated fatty acids also have the potential for causing diarrhea. In addition, with no proven value, the animal fish oil–enriched diets are expensive—with a cost that is double that of comparable foods not fortified with fish oil.

■ Feeding Foods Containing Nucleotides

A Requirement for Nucleotides[18]

Most dietary nitrogen is in protein, with nitrogen being an important part of every amino acid. Nitrogen is also a part of nucleotides that are essential to biochemical operations of all cells. Nucleotides are necessary for the production, use, and storage of cellular energy. They form DNA and RNA structures necessary for the genetic code and cellular protein production. Some nucleotides are messengers for biochemical events, and they can be part of enzyme systems.

Nucleotides are necessary for normal intestinal structure and function, and they promote gastrointestinal healing. Cottage cheese, tofu and rice, or tapioca diets are low in nucleotides. Since there are no nutritional requirements established by the National Research Council for nucleotides in small animals, this does not represent a deficiency. Part of the reason for this is that the body synthesizes nucleotides. Their production is costly in terms of energy, however. Thus, if a diet contains nucleotides, it will be easier for an animal to maintain the functions with which they are involved.

Supplementing diets with nucleotides has proven effects to optimize gastrointestinal growth and regeneration. Animals with diarrhea or intestinal damage recover more quickly when fed diets containing nucleotides. Such diets provide nucleotide precursors for mucosal renewal and for improved mucosal circulation. These diets also can promote a most favorable intestinal bacterial population.

Nucleotides help maintain intestinal immune responses that are essential to prevent invasion by intestinal bacteria. This is most important for immunocompromised animals.

The liver is important for making and exporting nucleotides. If disease compromises liver function as well as that of the intestinal tract, the liver is unable to maintain this function. Dietary nucleotides help here in recovery of both hepatic and intestinal diseases.

Nucleotides Added to the Diet

The diet should be supplemented with nucleotides for an animal recovering from gastrointestinal disease. Red meats are higher in nucleotides than most other foods. However, meats are not included in the diets for dogs with gastrointestinal disease; many dogs will not recover when they are fed meat. Thus, it is necessary to add another source of nucleotides. Nonmeat sources include asparagus, cauliflower, beans, lentils, peas, mushrooms, and spinach. In dogs and cats, fish and poultry are acceptable sources. Chapter 8 has recipes supplemented with nucleotides. They include the cottage cheese or tofu and rice diets that are enriched with one kind of nucleotide, purines.

■ Feeding Foods Containing Polyamines[19]

Polyamines are small compounds made from a few select amino acids. Specific ones have unusual names, such as spermine, cadaverine, and putrescine. The intestinal mucosa (and other tissues in the body) manufactures them. The diet also supplies polyamines.

Polyamines promote growth and multiplication of cells. Specific effects of polyamines include the ability to promote hypertrophy and hyperplasia of the gastrointestinal mucosa, inhibit gastric acid secretion, promote ulcer healing, prevent development of experimentally induced ulceration, and induce intestinal maturation and the development of digestive enzyme activity.

Polyamine deficiency slows recovery in the diseased mucosa. With damage to the mucosa, fewer cells are available to produce polyamines. If the diet is deficient in polyamines, healing is even slower. Normal intestinal structure and function cannot return until the mucosa heals. Restoration of the mucosa takes about a week, and that requires optimal amounts of polyamines.

The diet should contain adequate polyamines and precursors for their formation. Soybean isolates are very high in polyamines. In contrast, milk protein–based diets are very low in polyamines. In Chapter

8, the diets containing tofu are high in polyamines, and the cottage cheese diets contain low amounts.

The digestive tract's requirement for polyamines is demonstrated through the use of inhibitors of polyamine formation. Such inhibitors are used to treat malignantly growing cells in the digestive system. Inhibitors reducing polyamine levels slow cancer cell growth and multiplication. Reducing dietary polyamine levels has the same effect.

Resting and Cleansing the Intestinal Tract[4]

With colonic contents containing many substances that can cause damage and inflammation, their removal would benefit in managing colonic disease. In the 1950s veterinarians frequently gave dogs enemas to treat acute digestive tract diseases. Giving large amounts caused fluid movement into the small intestine, and some was vomited. Giving enemas until dogs vomited was helpful but for reasons unknown at the time.

Animals with acute intestinal tract damage heal faster when intestinal contents are washed out. Both structure and function return to normal faster. Healing is slower when drugs are used to retain contents in the intestine. Motility modifiers such as loperamide cause such a retention.

Continued exposure of the injured intestinal mucosa to intestinal contents stimulates inflammation. Cleansing the intestine prevents inflammation, and any injury heals without being delayed by inflammation. Cleansing is the only way to remove bacteria and toxins such as endotoxins. Other substances, such as certain foods, are eliminated by not feeding commercial pet foods; nothing or a controlled diet is fed.

Intestinal Tract Healing Takes Time

When feeding is resumed for animals with intestinal damage, digestion remains abnormal until mucosal cells regain their ability to produce and secrete digestive enzymes. Animals lose that ability and do not regain it for five to seven days, the time necessary for renewal of the cells producing enzymes. Mucosal damage also impairs nutrient absorption; five to seven days are required for its recovery.

A great mistake made in caring for animals recovering from mucosal damage is to continue feeding commercial pet foods that are not adequately digested and absorbed. With incomplete assimilation, gut contents contain foods that can be absorbed and provoke allergies. Owners often wish to feed commercial pet foods after signs of gastrointestinal problems disappear. Commercial food should not be fed when an allergy to a food can develop. Unfortunately, recovery can appear to be complete long before the intestinal mucosa is normal. Diarrhea, vomiting, and inappetite disappear days before recovery is complete. Animals will usually beg for food at this time, and owners often give them what they want.

Summary

Care and feeding of animals with gastrointestinal problems, causing chronic diarrhea and sometimes persistent vomiting, require a protocol for the most favorable environment for healing. This protocol is based on selecting a diet that is optimally digested and absorbed. No drugs are given unless there are specific indications or dietary management fails. Healing requires management for at least a week before it is complete. With a food allergy it may require months before oral tolerance is regained. Continuing to feed offending foods, even in small amounts that cause no signs of diarrhea, will cause allergies to persist; tolerance for food is never regained.

References

1. Guilford, W. Grant. 1996. Gastrointestinal immune system. In *Strombeck's Small Animal Gastroenterology,* 2d ed., edited by W. Grant Guilford, Sharon A. Center, Donald R. Strombeck, David A. Williams, and Denny J. Meyer, 20–39. Philadelphia: W.B. Saunders.

2. Guilford, W. Grant. 1996. Gastrointestinal inflammation. In *Strombeck's Small Animal Gastroenterology,* 2d ed., edited by W. Grant Guilford, Sharon A. Center, Donald R. Strombeck, David A. Williams, and Denny J. Meyer, 40–49. Philadelphia: W.B. Saunders.

3. Boedeker, Edgar C. 1994. Adherent bacteria: Breaching the mucosal barrier? *Gastroenterology* 106(1):255–257.

4. Guilford, W. Grant and Donald R. Strombeck. 1996. Classification, pathophysiology, and symptomatic treatment of diarrheal diseases. In *Strombeck's Small Animal Gastroenterology,* 2d ed., edited by W. Grant Guilford, Sharon A. Center, Donald R. Strombeck, David A. Williams, and Denny J.

Meyer, 351–356. Philadelphia: W.B. Saunders.

5. Meyer, H. and E. Kienzle. 1991. Dietary protein and carbohydrates: Relationship to clinical disease. Purina International Nutrition Symposium in association with the Eastern States Veterinary Conference, January 15, Orlando, Florida, 13–26.

6. McArdle, A. Hope. 1994. Protection from radiation injury by elemental diet: Does added glutamine change the effect? *Gut* supplement 1:S60–S64.

7. Bauer, John E. and Ian E. Maskell. 1994. Dietary fibre: Perspectives in clinical management. In *The Waltham Book of Clinical Nutrition of the Dog and Cat*, edited by J.M. Wills and K.W. Simpson, 87–104. Oxford: Pergamon Press.

8. Deitch, E.A. 1994. Bacterial translocation: The influence of dietary variables. *Gut* supplement 1:S23–S27.

9. Ciancio, Mae J. 1994. Endotoxin-induced diarrhea in inflammatory bowel disease: Cellular and molecular mechanisms. *Progress Inflammatory Bowel Disease* 15(1):17.

10. Funk, Martha A. and David H. Baker. 1991. Effect of fiber, protein source and time of feeding on methotrexate toxicity in rats. *Journal of Nutrition* 121:1673–1683.

11. McArthur, K.E., J.H. Walsh, and C.T. Richardson. 1988. Soy protein meals stimulate less gastric acid secretion and gastrin release than beef meals. *Gastroenterology* 95:920–926.

12. Fernandez-Banares, F., E. Cabre, F. Gonzalez-Huix, and M.A. Gassull. 1994. Enteral nutrition as primary therapy in Crohn's disease. *Gut* supplement 1:S55–S59.

13. Drevon, Christian A. 1992. Marine oils and their effects. *Nutrition Reviews* 50(4):38–45.

14. Aw, T.Y., C.A. Rhoads, D.F. Smith, R. Iwakiri, and J.R. Zahn. 1994. Intestinal inflammation and oxidative stress are associated with fish oil feeding in the rat. *Gastroenterology* A647.

15. Vaughn, D.M., G.A. Reinhart, S.F. Swaim, S.D. Lauten, M.K. Boudreaux, J.S. Spano, and C. Hoffman. 1994. Evaluation of dietary N-6 to N-3 fatty acid ratios on leukotriene B synthesis in dog skin and neutrophils. *Journal of Veterinary Internal Medicine* 8(2):155.

16. Anonymous. 1994. New concepts in pruritic management. In *Topics in Practical Nutrition*. Dayton, Ohio: IAMS Company, 4:3.

17. Hanauer, Stephen B. 1994. Evolving medical therapies for inflammatory bowel disease. *Progress in Inflammatory Bowel Disease* 15:(2)1–5.

18. Grimble, G.K. 1994. Dietary nucleotides and gut mucosal defence. *Gut* supplement 1:S46–S51.

19. McCormack, Shirley A. and Leonard R. Johnson. 1991. Role of polyamines in gastrointestinal mucosal growth. *American Journal of Physiology* (Gastrointestinal Liver Physiology 23):G795–G806.

CHAPTER 10
Diet and Skin Disease

Incidence and Breed Distribution of Diet-Related Skin Disease[1-3]

Skin diseases are the most common problems treated by veterinarians. In quite a few areas of the country, they account for more than 50 percent of all the animals presented, both the normal and the abnormal, to a veterinary practice. Up to 10 percent of the dermatologic problems are due to dietary allergies. Food allergies are more likely in certain breeds of dog. Breeds more prone to food allergies than others include Labrador retrievers, cocker spaniels, collies, springer spaniels, and miniature schnauzers. Food allergies can appear at any age, with some animals showing clinical signs before they are a year old. Sometimes, an offending allergen is consumed for two years or longer before any clinical signs appear.

Causes of Diet-Related Skin Disease[1-3]

Few studies identify a cause of food-induced skin problems in dogs and cats. Veterinarians believe that dietary deficiencies are one cause because a few skin problems respond to treatment with nutrients such as zinc, vitamin A, vitamin B, vitamin E, protein, or some essential fatty acids.

Dietary hypersensitivity and food intolerance are more likely than a deficiency to cause skin disease. Food hypersensitivity or immune-mediated reactions develop in the same way that digestive tract problems do (see Chapters 6 and 7). Food intolerances develop when a dietary nonnutrient causes skin disease. A large number of dietary nonnutrient additives are listed in Chapter 3. How common are these cases of additive-related skin diseases? An expert states: "There are no definitive reports of adverse reactions to food additives in animals. However, many clinicians have seen cats that develop pruritic skin disease when fed any commercial diet and that are asymptomatic when fed homemade diets."[4]

Histamine is released during a hypersensitivity response to food. Some foods also contain histamine as a contaminant. Chemical breakdown of the amino acid histidine forms histamine. Bacteria can cause this reaction, and bacterial contamination of food can produce large amounts of histamine. Canned fish products are often high in histamine, reflecting bacterial contamination before canning. Dried and fermented foods (cheeses and meats) also contain high amounts of histamine. Some pet foods containing high histamine concentrations can cause skin problems.

Some foods can promote histamine release in humans. They include egg whites, shellfish, fish, chocolate, strawberries, and tomatoes. There is no evidence that these foods cause problems in dogs or cats, however.

Clinical Signs of Diet-Related Skin Disease[1-3]

Food allergies usually cause animals to be pruritic. The pruritus is associated with no external parasites and is nonseasonal. Many animals also have papules, and some show evidence of secondary staphylococcal skin infection. In one-half of the cases, the skin is markedly erythemic and shows signs of self-trauma. In long-standing cases seborrhea, hyperpigmentation, and lichenification are common. Atopy, one form of allergic skin disease a dietary allergen can cause, produces pruritus of the feet, face, ears, and underside of the body. Other forms of food allergies can affect any part of the body. Involvement of the ears results in otitis externa. Otitis externa is usually treated successfully with antibiotics. When otitis externa does not completely disappear or recurs after treatment stops, a food allergy should be suspected as the cause.

Diagnosis of Food Allergies[1-3]

The diagnosis of a food allergy can be difficult to prove. There are no laboratory tests to confirm a food allergy as the cause of either skin or gastrointestinal disease. Intradermal skin tests are often used to identify different allergens as the cause of skin disease. No studies have shown that skin testing for food allergens is reliable. This testing commonly produces false-positive reactions that lead to overestimates of the incidence of food allergies.

Testing for food allergies can also include radioallergosorbent tests (RAST) and enzyme-linked immunosorbent assays (ELISA). These tests detect antibodies against specific allergens, here, food allergens. No studies in dogs and cats prove any value for these tests.

Many chronic skin problems are evaluated with blood tests and skin biopsies. Complete blood counts and blood chemistry panels provide little useful information for identifying food allergies or intolerances. Skin biopsies never show changes that indicate food allergies. All changes found by biopsies are nonspecific, such as inflammation.

Dietary Management[1-3]

Feeding a controlled diet is the only long-term acceptable treatment for food allergies causing skin disease. A controlled diet is formulated to be balanced and free of allergens, most of which are proteins. The diet is made with ingredients most likely to be tolerated. Few studies prove that any one food is less likely than others to cause allergies.[5] Foods believed to be best tolerated include lamb, chicken, horse meat, venison, and rabbit because they are not usually found in commercial pet foods. Lack of exposure to these foods makes it less likely they would provoke an allergic response. One of these protein sources is combined with boiled rice or potatoes to form the only diet fed for at least three weeks. Chapter 8 lists many diets for managing gastrointestinal diseases that can be used for controlling skin diseases. Additional recipes follow.

Sometimes pruritus continues for months after offending foods are removed from the diet. Current recommendations are to feed a controlled diet for 60 days before making any conclusions about unexplained and persisting pruritus.

Many commercial diets are available for treating dietary allergies. Lamb and rice are usually their primary ingredients. They may not be effective, however. Pruritus and skin disease caused by dietary allergies often disappear when dogs eat lamb and rice diets prepared by owners. Skin problems return for some when they are fed a commercially prepared diet of lamb and rice. Other than vitamins and minerals, owner-prepared foods contain no other nutrients. Commercial diets contain fillers, additives, and preservatives that may be responsible for a relapse of an allergic skin disease.

An animal can be allergic to other preparations it consumes. Vitamin-mineral preparations contain meat products and additives to which an animal can be allergic. Signs of an allergy often return when a vitamin-mineral tablet or powder is added to balance a controlled diet. Medications given to prevent heartworms also contain additives that can cause signs of an allergy. These supplements are not given until a diagnosis of a food allergy can be confirmed. Adult animals show no signs of deficiency if vitamin and mineral supplements are not given for six to eight weeks. Hypoallergenic vitamin-mineral supplements can be given when more commonly used supplements cause signs of an allergy. Vitamin B_{12} should be given by tablet several times a month or by feeding a food such as sardines that contains abundant amounts.

Rabbit and Potato Diet for Adult Dogs

1/2 cup rabbit, cooked, diced

3 cups potato, boiled with skin

2 teaspoons vegetable (canola) oil

1/10 teaspoon table salt

4 bonemeal tablets (10-grain or equivalent)

1/5 multiple vitamin-mineral tablet (made for adult humans)

Provides 647 kilocalories, 29.3 grams protein, 17.6 grams fat
Supports caloric needs of a 20-pound dog

Venison and Potato Diet for Adult Dogs

4½ ounces venison (raw weight), cooked

3 cups potato, boiled with skin

2 teaspoons vegetable (canola) oil

¹/₁₀ teaspoon table salt

4 bonemeal tablets (10-grain or equivalent)

¹/₅ multiple vitamin-mineral tablet (made for adult humans)

Provides 656 kilocalories, 35.7 grams protein, 15.7 grams fat
Supports caloric needs of a 20-pound dog

Rabbit and Rice Diet for Adult Dogs

½ cup rabbit, cooked, diced

2 cups rice, long-grain, cooked

2 teaspoons vegetable (canola) oil

¹/₁₀ teaspoon table salt

4 bonemeal tablets (10-grain or equivalent)

¹/₅ multiple vitamin-mineral tablet (made for adult humans)

Provides 651 kilocalories, 29.2 grams protein, 18.2 grams fat
Supports caloric needs of a 20-pound dog

Venison and Rice Diet for Adult Dogs

4¹/₂ ounces venison (raw weight), cooked

2 cups rice, long-grain, cooked

2 teaspoons vegetable (canola) oil

¹/₄ teaspoon salt substitute—potassium chloride

¹/₁₀ teaspoon table salt

4 bonemeal tablets (10-grain or equivalent)

¹/₅ multiple vitamin-mineral tablet (made for adult humans)

Provides 660 kilocalories, 35.5 grams protein, 16.1 grams fat
Supports caloric needs of a 20- to 21-pound dog

Rabbit and Potato Diet for Growing Dogs

¹/₂ cup rabbit, cooked, diced

2 cups potato, boiled with skin

2 teaspoons vegetable (canola) oil

¹/₁₀ teaspoon table salt

4 bonemeal tablets (10-grain or equivalent)

¹/₅ multiple vitamin-mineral tablet (made for adult humans)

Provides 511 kilocalories, 26.4 grams protein, 17.4 grams fat
See Table 4.2 in Chapter 4 for a growing dog's caloric needs.

Venison and Potato Diet for Growing Dogs

4¹/₂ ounces (before cooking) venison, cooked

2 cups potatoes, boiled with skin

2 teaspoons vegetable (canola) oil

¹/₁₀ teaspoon table salt

4 bonemeal tablets (10-grain or equivalent)

¹/₅ multiple vitamin-mineral tablet (made for adult humans)

Provides 520 kilocalories, 32.7 grams protein, 15.5 grams fat
See Table 4.2 in Chapter 4 for a growing dog's caloric needs.

Rabbit and Rice Diet for Growing Dogs

¹/₂ cup rabbit, cooked, diced

1¹/₄ cups rice, long-grain, cooked

2 teaspoons vegetable (canola) oil

¹/₁₀ teaspoon table salt

4 bonemeal tablets (10-grain or equivalent)

¹/₅ multiple vitamin-mineral tablet (made for adult humans)

Provides 497 kilocalories, 26 grams protein, 17.8 grams fat
See Table 4.2 in Chapter 4 for a growing dog's caloric needs.

Venison and Rice Diet for Growing Dogs

4½ ounces (before cooking) venison, cooked

1¼ cups rice, long-grain, cooked

2 teaspoons vegetable (canola) oil

¼ teaspoon salt substitute—potassium chloride

¹/₁₀ teaspoon table salt

4 bonemeal tablets (10-grain or equivalent)

¹/₅ multiple vitamin-mineral tablet (made for adult humans)

Provides 506 kilocalories, 32.3 grams protein, 15.8 grams fat
See Table 4.2 in Chapter 4 for a growing dog's caloric needs.

Rabbit Diet for Adult or Growing Cats

¾ cup rabbit, cooked, diced

1 tablespoon vegetable (canola) oil

¼ teaspoon salt substitute—potassium chloride

2 bonemeal tablets (10-grain or equivalent)

¹/₁₀ multiple vitamin-mineral tablet (made for adult humans)

Provides 352 kilocalories, 31.1 grams protein, 25.1 grams fat
See Table 4.4 in Chapter 4 for a cat's or kitten's caloric needs.

Venison Diet for Adult or Growing Cats

4½ ounces venison (raw weight), cooked

4 teaspoons vegetable (canola) oil

¼ teaspoon salt substitute—potassium chloride

2 bonemeal tablets (10-grain or equivalent)

¹⁄₁₀ multiple vitamin-mineral tablet (made for adult humans)

Provides 331 kilocalories, 27.2 grams protein, 24.6 grams fat
See Table 4.4 in Chapter 4 for a cat's or kitten's caloric needs.

Rabbit and Potato Diet for Adult Cats

½ cup rabbit, cooked, diced

¾ cup potato, boiled with skin

1 tablespoon vegetable (canola) oil

¹⁄₁₀ teaspoon table salt

¼ teaspoon salt substitute—potassium chloride

2 bonemeal tablets (10-grain or equivalent)

¹⁄₁₀ multiple vitamin-mineral tablet (made for adult humans)

Provides 378 kilocalories, 23 grams protein, 21.6 grams fat
See Table 4.4 in Chapter 4 for a cat's or kitten's caloric needs.

Venison and Potato Diet for Adult Cats

3 ounces venison (raw weight), cooked

³/₄ cup potatoes, boiled with skin

1 tablespoon vegetable (canola) oil

¹/₁₀ teaspoon table salt

¹/₄ teaspoon salt substitute—potassium chloride

2 bonemeal tablets (10-grain or equivalent)

¹/₁₀ multiple vitamin-mineral tablet (made for adult humans)

Provides 334 kilocalories, 20.4 grams protein, 17.9 grams fat
See Table 4.4 in Chapter 4 for a cat's or kitten's caloric needs.

Rabbit and Rice Diet for Adult Cats

¹/₂ cup rabbit, cooked, diced

¹/₂ cup rice, long-grain, cooked

1 tablespoon vegetable (canola) oil

¹/₁₀ teaspoon table salt

¹/₄ teaspoon salt substitute—potassium chloride

2 bonemeal tablets (10-grain or equivalent)

¹/₁₀ multiple vitamin-mineral tablet (made for adult humans)

Provides 379 kilocalories, 22.8 grams protein, 21.6 grams fat
See Table 4.4 in Chapter 4 for a cat's or kitten's caloric needs.

Venison and Rice Diet for Adult Cats

3 ounces venison (raw weight), cooked

½ cup rice, long-grain, cooked

1 tablespoon vegetable (canola) oil

¹/₁₀ teaspoon table salt

¼ teaspoon salt substitute—potassium chloride

2 bonemeal tablets (10-grain or equivalent)

¹/₁₀ multiple vitamin-mineral tablet (made for adult humans)

Provides 335 kilocalories, 20.3 grams protein, 18 grams fat
See Table 4.4 in Chapter 4 for a cat's or kitten's caloric needs.

Management Failures

Clinical signs of food allergies develop from chemicals released in sensitized individuals. Mostly, chemicals are released only after leukocytes interact with a food allergen. When the allergen disappears, the release of these chemicals stops. Sometimes, the chemicals continue to be released spontaneously without the allergen. The spontaneous chemical release may take months to decline and stop. In this case the animal can continue to show clinical signs of an allergy though the allergen is no longer fed. This is often mistakenly believed to be a treatment failure and one where the allergen is unknown. Patience is important in the dietary management of animals with food allergies.

References

1. Harvey, Richard G. 1994. Skin disease. In *The Waltham Book of Clinical Nutrition of the Dog and Cat*, edited by J.M. Wills and K.W. Simpson, 425–444. Oxford: Pergamon Press.

2. Halliwell, Richard E.W. 1992. *Dietary Hypersensitivity in the Dog*. A monograph. Vernon, Calif.: Kal Kan.

3. Wills, Josephine M. and Richard E.W. Halliwell. 1994. Dietary sensitiv-

ity. In *The Waltham Book of Clinical Nutrition of the Dog and Cat*, edited by J.M. Wills and K.W. Simpson, 167–188. Oxford: Pergamon Press.

4. Halliwell, Richard E.W. 1992. Comparative aspects of food intolerance. *Veterinary Medicine*, September, 893–899.

5. Jeffers, James G., Evelyn K. Meyer, and Ellen J. Sosis. 1996. Responses of dogs with food allergies to single-ingredient dietary provocation. *Journal of American Veterinary Medical Association* 209(3):608–611.

PART FOUR
Diet-Induced Disease

CHAPTER 11
Feeding to Manage Obesity

Obesity is the most common form of malnutrition affecting dogs in Western countries. Estimates suggest that up to 45 percent of dogs and up to 13 percent of cats in these countries are obese. Obesity can be judged from normal weight ranges published for purebred dogs. Normal ranges for a breed depend on height and conformation, so subjective evaluation is needed for deciding where an individual falls in its range. Many owners of definitely overweight animals believe their pets' weight to be "just right." Because obesity develops gradually, these owners cannot objectively evaluate their pets' condition. Current recommendations are to begin a weight management program if a pet is 15 percent or more over its ideal weight.

Causes of Obesity[1-3]

■ Gender and Breed Influences

People offer many causes for obesity. Female dogs and cats are believed more likely to be obese than male dogs and cats. There is no evidence for gender being a primary factor, however. Neutering is a cause, but obesity is secondary to neutering. Reduced physical activity, caused by the neutering, is the primary cause. There may be a greater tendency for obesity in some dog breeds. However, no scientific studies support that. Other factors believed to predispose an animal to obesity include older age, feeding owner-prepared foods, having an obese owner, and having a middle-aged or elderly owner. These factors all relate to food intake and physical activity. The primary cause of obesity is intake exceeding expenditure of energy, too much food, and too little exercise.

■ Metabolic Diseases

In some dogs (less than 5 percent) the cause of obesity is an endocrine disease such as hypothyroidism, hypogonadism, insulin deficiency or excess, and hyperadrenocorticism. The possibility of endocrine causes means physical examinations and laboratory evaluations must be conducted before obesity is managed.

■ Juvenile and Adult Bases of Obesity

The physiological basis varies for different forms of obesity. Increased food intake causing obesity in adults promotes fat accumulation in existing adipose cells. The numbers of fat cells do not increase; they merely enlarge. Overfeeding during growth increases fat cell numbers. Weight reduction is more difficult with increased numbers of fat cells than with increased fat in a normal number of cells. Thus, growing animals must not be overfed. Recommendations for feeding commercial pet food result in young animals being overfed. Larger size dogs should be fed 15 to 20 percent less food than recommended. This reduction also lessens orthopedic problems associated with overfeeding.

■ Satisfying Appetites

Today, the world tells people to "go for it" and to not deny any of their wants. Why shouldn't all members of a family, including the pets, be recipients of that advice? The pet food industry teaches us to give our pets foods that taste good—not to deny them the pleasures of life. The pet food industry's primary goal is to produce a food the animal will like better than any competitor's. Television commercials show how well dogs or cats consume the foods being advertised.

Is Obesity OK or Not OK?

When obesity results from owners indulging pets, the owners will not present the pets for treatment of obesity. Of pets examined for obesity (including those examined only after veterinarians compel owners to acknowledge the problem), most will not remain under treatment. Of those that remain under treatment, most will not lose weight. Of those that lose weight, most will regain it. For owners, an unacceptable medical problem is the most convincing reason to manage obesity. Many medical problems are not resolved without a weight loss.

Obesity's Effects on Health[1-3]

One of the most common medical problems caused or aggravated by obesity is arthritis. There are many drugs for management of arthritis. At best they are of temporary value. Aspirin continues to be effective, with few side effects in dogs. Newer nonsteroidal antiinflammatory drugs injure the gastrointestinal mucosa. If drugs are ineffective, a pet's weight must be reduced to manage arthritis. Owners will do this when they recognize that only weight reduction can help and that untreated obesity can shorten life span.

Additional medical problems associated with obesity in dogs include orthopedic problems such as herniated intervertebral discs and ruptured stifle ligaments. Obese animals also have difficulty breathing and maintaining normal circulation, and breathing and circulatory abnormalities aggravate heat intolerance. Obese pets are more likely to have diabetes mellitus and skin problems. Surgery is more difficult in obese animals, and they heal with more complications. Obese animals are also more likely to develop complications from or reactions to anesthesia.

Despite these problems owners are not likely to reduce their pets' weight. The exception is likely to be the result of orthopedic problems causing lameness. Owners are forced to do something; the problem is unacceptable.

Evaluation and Management of Obesity[1-3]

Success in weight reduction is possible with effective client education. Often little education is given. Obese pets are weighed and examined, and owners are sold a prescription diet formulated for weight reduction. (Although millions of dollars are spent on prescription diets annually, few of these diets have had any clinical trials to prove their claims.) A prescription diet is not likely to be successful for weight reduction unless owners understand what to expect. Client education is more important than any diet. Furthermore, prescription diets are not necessary for weight reduction: pet owners can prepare effective diets.

■ Evaluation of the Obese Animal

Obese animals should have a complete medical checkup before any weight control management is begun. Included should be a record of the pet's history and a physical examination. The physical determines whether ribs and the dorsal spine are easily felt. The size of lumbar and lower abdominal fat pads are examined. Presence of a waist and folds of fat in the cervical and other areas are noted.

Laboratory tests are used to identify the 5 percent of animals with medical problems causing obesity. Included are a complete blood count and chemistry panel. Usually, no other laboratory tests are needed.

■ Management of Obesity

Management of and client education about obesity should be based on the following protocol. The protocol includes five steps that are simple and easy to comprehend. The protocol is essential for successful weight reduction.

1. Estimate the pet's normal or optimal body weight or determine it through tables listing normal weights for the breed.

2. Knowing the pet's current body weight and the normal or optimal weight, calculate the body weight to be lost. Loss of body weight will occur only when energy intake is less than expenditure.

3. Calculate the calories in the body fat that must be lost. The amount to be lost equals the sum of daily calorie deficits that can be achieved. Calories lost or burned from fat equal the difference between calories consumed and calories expended as energy.

4. Estimate the calories to feed based on the pet's normal, not current, weight. The number of calories burned for energy depends on the size of muscle mass. For practical purposes, assume that only muscle burns nutrients for energy. Muscle mass is small in an obese animal. Feeding caloric requirements for normal, nonobese weights does not result in weight loss, however. Therefore, animals are fed no more than 50 percent of requirements based on normal body weight.

5. Calculate how many pounds should be lost each week. Weigh the pet weekly to ensure that the estimations are correct for the necessary caloric intake. Also, check that there is compliance by all family members who could feed the animal.

■ **Calculations for a Reducing Program**

To calculate the amount of food to feed in a weight reduction program, calculate the following:

A. Current body weight (in pounds) = _____
B. Desired body weight (in pounds) = _____
C. Body weight loss to achieve B (A − B) = _____
D. Kilocalories to lose (C × 3500) = _____
E. Energy requirements for normal weight
   Use a table identifying normal weight for the breed or use
   the formula 125 × (normal weight in kg)$^{0.75}$ = _____
F. Energy required to reduce weight
   (one-half E) = _____
   (Energy level of food should be 50 percent of needs.)
G. Energy obtained from burning of animal
   fat stores in one week (7 × F) = _____
H. Pounds of fat to be lost each week
   (G ÷ 3500) = _____
I. Weeks needed to lose excess fat
   (C ÷ H) = _____

To feed at the level identified by F, the energy required to reduce weight, it is necessary to know or to calculate the number of calories to be fed in the diet. Commercial pet food labels do not show the number of calories per pound, can, or cup of food. Thus, it is necessary to calculate the number of calories by using information found on the pet food label or to call the manufacturer for that information. Calculations should be based on the minimum amount of fat and the maximum amount of ash and moisture, as listed on the label, to approximate metabolizable energy (kilocalories) per ounce of any pet food. The calculations are as follows:

1. Add the percentages of fat, moisture, and ash. If the label does not list the ash percentage, use the figures 2.4 (canned meat), 3.1 (canned meat and cereal), 4.7 (semimoist food), 8.4 (dry food), or 9.6 (dry "high-protein" foods).
2. Subtract the total of number 1 from 100.
3. Add the figure from number 2 to 2.5 times the fat percentage. The sum equals the calories in each ounce of food.
4. Divide the sum from F by the sum from number 3 to calculate how many ounces of food to feed each day.

For example, Table 11.1 can be used to calculate the following:

1. Add percent of fat, moisture, and ash: 7 + 75 + 4 = 86.
2. Subtract number 1 from 100: 100 − 86 = 14.
3. Multiply the fat percent by 2.5: 7 × 2.5 = 17.5.
4. Add number 3 to that of number 2: 17.5 + 14 = 31.5 kilocalories per ounce.

Owner-prepared pet foods can also be fed. To do so requires comprehensive tables listing the caloric content of food ordinarily eaten by humans that animals can eat. This has been done for all the recipes in this book. Any of the recipes in the chapter on feeding a normal dog or cat (Chapter 5) can be used.

Example of Calculations for Weight Reduction in an Obese Dog

A. The dog's current body weight = 55 pounds
B. The dog's ideal body weight = 44 pounds
C. Body weight loss to achieve B = 11 pounds
D. Kilocalories to lose = 38,500 kilocalories
E. Energy needs for 44-pound condition = 1248 kilocalories per day
F. Energy required to reduce weight = 624 kilocalories per day
G. Energy from fat burned weekly = 4368 kilocalories per week
H. Pounds of fat to be lost per week = 1.248 pounds
I. Number of weeks to reach normal weight = 8.8 weeks

If a fortified canned meat diet is fed, the dog will receive 31.5 kilocalories per ounce of food. Multiply this by 19.8 ounces of food for a total of 624 kilocalories per day. Most canned dog foods contain approximately one pound of food. Thus, the dog will eat a little more than a can of food daily.

Table 11.1. Guaranteed analysis of canned fortified meat diet (example)

Nutrients	Percent
Fat	7.0
Ash	4.0
Moisture	75.0

Requirements for a Reducing Program to be Successful[1-3]

Reducing a pet's weight is easier said than done. Eating habits developed over a lifetime are usually difficult to change, for the pet and for us. "Habit is habit, and not to be flung out of the window by any man, but coaxed downstairs a step at a time" was observed by Mark Twain many years ago. A pet will try everything it can to convince the owner-feeder that it is being subjected to the cruelest punishment possible with the weight reduction program.

■ Changing Eating Habits

Success for a weight reduction program depends on the owner recognizing that a complex and well-established routine of habits must change, and they will not change easily overnight. Everyone involved must understand the behavior that has to change. Pet owners must be involved in planning any reducing program for which they will be responsible. The entire family must be involved for the program to be successful. Changes in a pet's and family's habits must also be realistic. As noted earlier, obesity prevails because pets become inactive. Their activity reflects family members' activity. If possible, family members should exercise the pet. Of course, that is realistic only if there is someone willing and able to do this. If an infirm or elderly owner can't exercise a pet, it is unrealistic to believe that the pet's activity will increase. Also, the pet may be inactive because it has health problems that would make exercise hazardous to its well-being.

Restriction of food intake may appear severe. Reducing caloric needs by half will cause pets to use every means possible for coaxing owners into feeding what they want. Feeding more than the recommended amount slows and may prevent weight reduction.

■ Muscle Burns Calories

Muscle tissue burns calories, and the amount of muscle usually is the same in a normal weight dog as it is when it gains 10 to 30 pounds of fat. Muscle mass grows only with increased physical activity, which can increase caloric requirements. Each additional pound of muscle can burn 60 calories a day.

It is essential that all caloric calculations be based on estimations of the animal's normal weight. The nature of the diet is not that important for weight reduction. Only the caloric content of the total daily intake is important.

Weight Reduction Programs

Any complete and balanced diet can be fed in a weight reduction program. Success is less likely if the diet that resulted in obesity remains unchanged. Feeding a low-calorie prescription type of diet may be helpful. Such diets are low in fat and high in fiber so that an ounce of food contains 20 percent (or more) fewer calories. Larger volumes are consumed to gain a given number of calories. Distention of the digestive system by food curbs appetite. Any low-caloric-density diet accomplishes that.

"Filling animals up" with low-calorie and high-fiber foods does little to satisfy most obese pets. They continue to beg for more and other foods. Dietary fiber reduces digestion and absorption, which reduces the calories used. Commercial pet foods prepared for special uses, such as weight reduction, are expensive, and they offer little advantage over any other diet.

■ Low-Calorie Owner-Prepared Diets

Diets planned and prepared by the owners are more likely to be successful in reducing weight. Low-calorie foods can be especially selected and fed to the animal. A dog can virtually eat anything humans eat. Vegetables and some fruits are consumed by many dogs. They provide few calories because dogs don't chew and grind their food as people do, so less nutrition (calories) is provided. Foods like lettuce are often a welcomed treat that stops a pet from begging. Lettuce is practically void of calories when eaten without salad dressing.

It is easy to prepare diets for dogs and cats. Their nutritional requirements are similar to people's. Humans don't have to rely on purchasing and eating "complete and balanced" commercial foods to be nutritionally satisfied. They choose to eat foods that are needed to remain healthy. Veterinarians have experience with many dogs and cats that eat diets prepared by their owners. Signs of deficiencies are rare. Sometimes a single food such as meat or liver is eaten, and signs of deficiency should appear, but they don't. Owner-prepared diets could need added vitamins and minerals. No studies show that animals on weight reduction programs require any such additions.

■ Feeding Foods to Minimize Fat Deposition

All foods contain calories, but not all are converted equally to fat. Many of the calories burned daily are for processing of a meal. That amount can be greater than the energy expended in muscle activity. During processing of dietary fat, only 2 percent of its calories are needed for its deposition in adipose tissue. The body needs more calories to convert dietary protein and carbohydrates to fats for storage. About 25 percent of the calories in these foods are burned for their conversion to and storage as fat. Thus, feeding a diet containing fat that has the same number of calories as a diet containing proteins and carbohydrates results in greater fat deposition. Feeding fat is more likely to make a pet fat.

Fewer calories convert to fat when an animal's metabolic rate increases. Omega-3 fatty acids increase metabolic rate so more energy is burned. These fatty acids are abundant in fish and some vegetable oils such as flaxseed. Omega-3 fatty acids are also available as a supplement from health food sources.

Other foods that increase metabolism include vegetables, whole grains, legumes, and fruits. They are rich in fiber, which slows digestion and absorption, resulting in more stable blood glucose.[4] Fluctuating blood glucose resulting in periodic high levels stimulates the release of hormones that promote fat production and storage. Fiber also binds lipolytic enzymes and fats themselves, thereby reducing fat absorption. Fiber increases intestinal transit, which also reduces fat absorption.

Metabolic processes require vitamins and minerals. Providing these nutrients ensures optimal metabolic rates for burning calories. Humans supplement their diets with chromium, which helps the body to lose fat and retain muscle tissue. Chromium is proven effective for this purpose in pets. Some amino acids are essential for proper fat metabolism. Methionine and lysine are needed to make carnitine, which is needed to carry fatty acids into mitochondria, where they are metabolized. Inadequate carnitine causes more fat to be stored than metabolized.

Some spices such as ginger, cayenne pepper, and mustard increase metabolism in humans. Little is known about their effects in pets. Such spices can be used if they cause no clinical problems.

Some novel nutrients may be useful in weight reduction. Citric acid is found in citrus fruits. Hydroxycitric acid is a similar compound found in the rind of a small tropical fruit people in Southern Asia have valued for centuries. This substance can curb appetite, increase metabolism, and inhibit fat synthesis. It is available in health food stores.

■ Establishing a Feeding Schedule

One person should be designated to measure (weighing is the most accurate way to measure) the entire daily amount to feed, and this person should do the feeding. The animal is fed alone (not with other dogs or cats) in two feedings. Twice-a-day feeding often satisfies better than a single feeding. More frequent feeding may be more beneficial. Eating very small meals minimizes conversion of carbohydrates and proteins into fat. Fasting followed by gorging promotes fat gain. No treats, whether they are leftovers or biscuits, are fed unless their caloric contents are calculated to determine they do not exceed the daily caloric allowance. Obese pets should be excluded from areas where family meals are prepared or eaten.

Neighbors and houseguests should be advised of a pet's dietary restrictions and that they are important for health reasons. Also, a pet's environment should be monitored. It is not possible to control the diet of a pet having unrestricted freedom in the neighborhood; it is not difficult for it to find food.

■ Weighing a Pet to Monitor Progress

Pets should be weighed periodically during the weight reduction program. Throughout their lives, all dogs and cats should be weighed weekly or monthly so that owners can recognize any changes. Frequently, owners will not recognize changes in body weight until they are marked. During weight reduction, losses may appear small, but a weight loss of one pound per week for a medium or large size dog is a sign of success. An animal should be weighed at the same time every day because its weight can vary throughout the day. Weighing can be done in the morning before feeding. The pet's weight should be recorded on a calendar.

■ Exercise and Weight Reduction

Control of food intake is essential for reduction, but because physical inactivity is an important cause of weight gain, knowledge about exercise and weight control can help in a weight reduction program.

However, increasing energy expenditure by promoting exercise is not an easy way to reduce body weight. Exercise as an adjunct to weight reduction has some psychological value to the pet owner but, alone, will do little for the pet. For both an obese, aged dog with respiratory and cardiac problems and an aged or infirm owner, increased exercise could even be dangerous. Also, obese animals are generally reluctant to exercise, although there can be some success when their owners run or jog regularly. If an animal's weight reduction and maintenance program is to include exercise, it should begin after the pet has lost most of its excess weight. It may be helpful to note that people who walk more than 30 minutes each day for at least a year can lose 10 to 40 pounds without any dietary restrictions.

■ Drugs for Weight Reduction

Many people would like to reduce weight for their obese pets by giving medication rather than following any dietary restrictions or increasing exercise. No such medications are effective for weight reduction in dogs or cats. Drugs used but ineffective include amphetamines to reduce appetite, thyroid hormones to increase metabolism, tranquilizers, and diuretics.

■ Starvation for Weight Reduction

The fastest way to reduce weight is by starvation. Complete starvation reduces body weight to approximately 75 percent of prestarvation weight within five to six weeks (Fig. 11.1). The 55-pound dog in the earlier example should lose 14 pounds to drop to 75 percent of its weight. If nothing is eaten, the dog should lose about a third of a pound a day. In one week it would lose about 2.5 pounds and in five weeks 12.5 pounds. Studies verify such losses with starvation.[5]

Owners could not starve a pet for four to six weeks. Furthermore, starvation cannot be justified. Regulatory branches of the government, which oversee animal experiments to ensure humane treatment, judge starvation of dogs, cats, or other animals as inhumane. Starving a pet is not the same as a human starving for weight reduction. A person can make the choice; the animal cannot.

A pet could be starved if it is hospitalized. Few adverse effects would be recognized. People who starve to lose weight develop medical complications from rapid catabolism of excess fat. Although complications are not recognized in dogs, blood glucose decreases, prod-

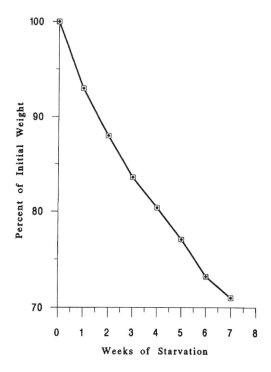

Figure 11.1. Weight loss during starvation (adapted from Morris, 1995).

ucts of incomplete fat metabolism increase, and the liver accumulates fat. Despite that, some studies on dogs starved for three to six weeks report no adverse clinical or biochemical changes.[5] Because some significant changes can occur during complete starvation, it should not be used to manage obesity in dogs.

Starvation may succeed in reducing weight during hospitalization for five to six weeks, but it will be expensive. More importantly, pets may readily regain the lost weight when they return home. This is likely because the owners were not involved with the "pangs" of weight reduction. These owners learned no compelling reasons for changing the lifelong habits that led to obesity; they will not fully appreciate the changes essential to prevent regain of lost weight. People who suffer through weight loss find it nearly impossible to change their habits and prevent a regain of lost weight. When owners know even less about what is involved in their pets' obesity problems, it will be even more difficult to prevent a regain of lost weight.

Obesity in Cats

Cats are often obese but not with the frequency seen in dogs. Cats probably can regulate food intake better than dogs, so fewer become obese. The weight of obese cats can be reduced, but this requires greater monitoring because they are more prone to developing complications. When a cat stops eating, fat accumulates in the liver within one week, and by two weeks the situation is invariably pathological. That is in contrast to the dog, for which starvation for five to six weeks has a less adverse effect. Accumulation of fat in the liver results in hepatic lipidosis. Affected cats stop eating and quickly develop jaundice. Without immediate treatment they die, often within days. Whenever a cat is presented by an owner who knows it hasn't eaten for more than one week, the animal should be tube fed as the first and most important step. That should be done before any diagnostic tests are performed. Problems with hepatic lipidosis are more serious than most other problems that the cat could have.

Weight Reduction Diets for Dogs

The following diets are low-fat and high-protein, and some are high-carbohydrate. They contain more fiber than maintenance diets. Vegetables are added for the additional fiber. Table 4.1 in Chapter 4 should be used to determine how many calories a dog requires when its body weight is normal. Half that amount is fed to obese dogs.

Each recipe gives caloric content and for what size dog that amount would be appropriate. A given dog is not likely to weigh the amount that each recipe or half a recipe is designed for. Increase or decrease the portions in a recipe to meet a pet's needs. Recipes can be made in large batches and divided into portions for meeting a pet's needs. Diets can be refrigerated or frozen in portions needed for one day. Daily portions can be heated or warmed to room temperature before feeding.

To illustrate how much to feed each day, imagine that an overweight dog weighs 35 pounds and should weigh 25 pounds. Using Table 4.1, the daily caloric requirements for adult dogs, in Chapter 4, you can estimate that a 25-pound dog should eat 772 kilocalories a day. Reduce this by one-half (386 kilocalories) to determine how much the obese dog should consume. The following chicken and boiled rice diet provides 624 kilocalories. Therefore, feed only about 60 percent of this amount. If the amounts in this diet are tripled so that its total calories are 1872, it will feed the 25-pound dog for about five days (1872 divided by 386).

As another example one batch of the chicken and rice diet, containing 624 kilocalories, provides for the reduced caloric needs of an obese dog that should weight 7 to 8 pounds for four days.

■ Vegetable Supplements

To each of the following diets, vegetables can be added. They are not necessary, but their addition should help satisfy a pet's appetite. The number of calories added with the inclusion of vegetables is found in Table 5.1. Uncooked vegetables contain few available calories, so if they are included or fed as snacks, it is not important to calculate their caloric contribution to the pet's intake. They provide additional fiber.

Commercial fiber preparations can be added to the diet. Claims are made that fiber helps to curb an animal's appetite, but that has not been proven. Examples of fiber that can be added include wheat bran and forms of cellulose. A medium size dog (25 to 40 pounds) can be given one to two heaping teaspoons of fiber in its food daily. If the amount greatly increases the volume of feces, reduce the fiber given. If fiber supplementation has no effect on satisfying the animal's appetite, there is no good reason to continue giving fiber.

■ Weight Reduction Diets for Adult Dogs

Chicken and Rice Diet

½ pound chicken (raw weight), cooked

2 cups rice, long-grain, cooked

¼ teaspoon salt substitute—potassium chloride

¹⁄₁₀ teaspoon table salt

4 bonemeal tablets

1 multiple vitamin-mineral tablet

Provides 624 kilocalories, 49.4 grams protein, 4.7 grams fat

Supplies the daily caloric needs for weight reduction in a dog normally 47 to 48 pounds (nonobese weight). One-half of this recipe supplies the daily caloric needs for weight reduction in a dog normally 19 pounds.

Chicken and Potato Diet

½ pound chicken (raw weight), cooked

3 cups potato, cooked with skin

⅒ teaspoon table salt

4 bonemeal tablets (10-grain or equivalent)

1 multiple vitamin-mineral tablet

Provides 620 kilocalories, 49.6 grams protein, 4.7 grams fat
Supplies the daily caloric needs for weight reduction in a dog normally 47 pounds (nonobese weight). One-half of this recipe supplies the caloric needs for weight reduction in a dog normally 19 pounds.

Egg Whites and Potato Diet

Egg whites from 4 eggs, hard-boiled

3 cups potato, cooked with skin

½ teaspoon vegetable (canola) oil

4 bonemeal tablets (10-grain or equivalent)

1 multiple vitamin-mineral tablet

Provides 491 kilocalories, 22.4 grams protein, 2.8 grams fat
Supplies the daily caloric needs for weight reduction in a dog normally 34 to 35 pounds (nonobese weight). One-half of this recipe supplies the caloric needs for weight reduction in a dog normally 13 to 14 pounds.

Egg Whites and Rice Diet

Egg whites from 4 eggs, hard-boiled

2 cups rice, long-grain, cooked

½ teaspoon vegetable (canola) oil

4 bonemeal tablets (10-grain or equivalent)

1 multiple vitamin-mineral tablet

Provides 495 kilocalories, 22.2 grams protein, 3.2 grams fat

Supplies the daily caloric needs for weight reduction in a dog normally 34 to 35 pounds (nonobese weight). One-half of this recipe supplies the caloric needs for weight reduction in a dog normally 13 to 14 pounds.

Cottage Cheese and Boiled Rice Diet

½ cup cottage cheese, 1 percent fat

2 cups rice, long-grain, cooked

½ teaspoon vegetable (canola) oil

¼ teaspoon salt substitute—potassium chloride

4 bonemeal tablets (10-grain or equivalent)

1 multiple vitamin-mineral tablet

Provides 512 kilocalories, 22.6 grams protein, 4.3 grams fat

Supplies the daily caloric needs for weight reduction in a dog normally 36 to 37 pounds (nonobese weight). One-half of this recipe supplies the caloric needs for weight reduction in a dog normally 14 to 15 pounds.

Cottage Cheese and Potato Diet

½ *cup cottage cheese, 1 percent fat*

3 cups potato, cooked with skin

½ *teaspoon vegetable (canola) oil*

4 bonemeal tablets (10-grain or equivalent)

1 multiple vitamin-mineral tablet

Provides 508 kilocalories, 22.8 grams protein, 3.9 grams fat

Supplies the daily caloric needs for weight reduction in a dog normally 36 to 37 pounds (nonobese weight). One-half of this recipe supplies the caloric needs for weight reduction in a dog normally 14 to 15 pounds.

Weight Reduction Diets for Cats

An owner must be more careful when reducing a cat's weight than a dog's. The caloric requirements of cats should be met at a level of no less than 60 percent of normal (normal caloric intake can be found in Table 4.4). Feeding less can result in a cat developing hepatic lipidosis. It occurs most frequently in obese cats that suddenly stop eating, sometimes for only a week. The following diets provide 60 percent of a cat's calories based on its normal body weight.

The diets do not contain any beef, lamb, or fish such as sardines because each is high in fat. High amounts of fat are not detrimental because of a risk for causing fatty liver, however. The fat content should be low in reducing diets for cats so most of the calories they consume contain the high amounts of protein they require.

Cats usually do not choose to eat vegetables. They are not necessary. It is also not necessary to supplement their diets with fiber.

Salmon Diet

5 ounces salmon, canned with bone (low-salt)

½ calcium carbonate tablet (200 milligrams calcium)

½ multiple vitamin-mineral tablet (made for pets)

Provides 215 kilocalories, 28.8 grams protein, 10.2 grams fat

Supplies the daily caloric needs for weight reduction in a cat that normally weighs 11 pounds. For a cat that normally weighs 9 to 10 pounds, feed 80 to 90 percent of the amount in this recipe.

Salmon and Rice Diet

5 ounces salmon, canned with bone (low-salt)

⅓ cup rice, long-grain, cooked

½ calcium carbonate tablet (200 milligrams calcium)

½ multiple vitamin-mineral tablet

Provides 284 kilocalories, 30.2 grams protein, 10.4 grams fat

Feed 75 percent of this recipe to a cat that normally weighs 11 pounds, 67 percent to a cat that normally weighs 10 pounds, and 60 percent to a cat that normally weighs 9 pounds.

Tuna Diet

8 ounces tuna, canned in water, without added salt

1 teaspoon vegetable (canola) oil

2 bonemeal tablets (10-grain or equivalent)

½ multiple vitamin-mineral tablet

Provides 290 kilocalories, 53.8 grams protein, 9.1 grams fat

Feed 75 percent of this recipe to a cat that normally weighs 11 pounds, 67 percent to a cat that normally weighs 10 pounds, and 60 percent to a cat that normally weighs 9 pounds.

Tuna and Rice Diet

4 ounces tuna, canned in water, without added salt

⅓ cup rice, long-grain, cooked

½ teaspoon vegetable (canola) oil

1 bonemeal tablet (10-grain or equivalent)

½ multiple vitamin-mineral tablet

Provides 219 kilocalories, 30.1 grams protein, 3.4 grams fat
Feed 100 percent of this recipe to a cat that normally weighs
11 pounds, 90 percent to a cat that normally weighs 10 pounds,
and 80 percent to a cat that normally weighs 9 pounds.

Chicken Diet

½ pound boneless chicken breast (raw weight), cooked

2 bonemeal tablets (10-grain or equivalent)

½ multiple vitamin-mineral tablet

Provides 239 kilocalories, 45.8 grams protein, 4.8 grams fat
Feed 100 percent of this recipe to a cat that normally weighs
11 pounds, 90 percent to a cat that normally weighs 10 pounds,
and 80 percent to a cat that normally weighs 9 pounds.

Chicken and Rice Diet

½ pound boneless chicken breast (raw weight), cooked

⅓ cup rice, long-grain, cooked

¼ teaspoon salt substitute—potassium chloride

2 bonemeal tablets (10-grain or equivalent)

½ multiple vitamin-mineral tablet

Provides 308 kilocalories, 47.2 grams protein, 5.1 grams fat
Feed 75 percent of this recipe to a cat that normally weighs

11 pounds, 67 percent to a cat that normally weighs 10 pounds, and 60 percent to a cat that normally weighs 9 pounds.

Low-Calorie Dog Biscuits or Treats

Recipes for dog biscuits can be found in Chapter 5. Caloric content is given, and biscuits can be fed as "treats," but the calories fed must be within the daily caloric allowance for the pet.

Summary

An understanding of what to expect in reducing the weight of an obese animal is essential for success. Living patterns must be changed for both owners and their pets. Calculations must be made on how many calories a pet needs. It is also necessary to understand how much weight an animal can lose each week. Weight reduction is a slow process. No dramatic losses of weight should be expected. Owners can prepare effective weight reduction diets for their pets. More care is necessary for reducing the weight of an obese cat than an obese dog.

References

1. Markwell, Peter J. and Richard F. Butterwick. 1994. Obesity. In *The Waltham Book of Clinical Nutrition of the Dog and Cat*, edited by J.M. Wills and K.W. Simpson, 131–148. Oxford: Pergamon Press.

2. Edney, A.T.B. and P.M. Smith. 1986. Study of obesity in dogs visiting veterinary practices in the United Kingdom. *Veterinary Record* 118:391–396.

3. Wolfsheimer, Karen J. Obesity in dogs. 1994. *Compendium Continuing Education Practicing Veterinarian* 16:981–998.

4. Bauer, John E. and Ian E. Maskell. 1994. Dietary fibre: Perspectives in clinical management. In *The Waltham Book of Clinical Nutrition of the Dog and Cat*, edited by J.M. Wills and K.W. Simpson, 87–104. Oxford: Pergamon Press.

5. Morris, James G. 1995. *Nutrition and Nutritional Diseases in Animals*. 5-1 to 5-9. Class Notes for Veterinary Medicine 408, School of Veterinary Medicine, University of California, Davis.

CHAPTER 12
Diet-Related Skeletal and Joint Diseases in Dogs

People purchase dogs for quite a lot of different reasons. For companionship it is much less expensive and less troublesome to own a small size than a large breed dog. Ownership of a large breed dog usually offers people a more athletic pet that can also fill an image of the type of dog an owner wants. Often puppies are selected with the hope they will mature into the biggest dogs for their breeds. Owners select the largest puppies in litters and ask for feeding advice to ensure growth. They will feed whatever it takes to gain the desired size. If everything is done to satisfy these owners' wants, it is very likely that their animals will develop one or more orthopedic problems.[1] Diseases of the joints and skeleton are often serious problems in large and giant breed dogs.

Diseases Caused by Overnutrition[1-3]

Hip dysplasia has been and continues to be very common, accounting for nearly one-third of all orthopedic cases seen by veterinarians. This degenerative joint disease results in a shallow acetabulum and flattened femoral head. The hip joint is partially luxated and shows secondary arthritis. Hip dysplasia occurs in 1 out of 60 dogs of all sizes. The risk in giant and large breed dogs is 20 to 50 times more likely than in others. Overnutrition is a major cause.

Many dogs with hip disease have problems in other bones and joints. One of these problems is hypertrophic osteodystrophy, which by definition means excessive nutrition resulting in bone malnutrition. Bony changes cause lameness, and affected bones are hot and painful. Excessive intake of protein, energy, calcium, and phosphorus accelerates growth and induces the problem.

Osteochrondosis dissecans is characterized by a discontinuity between the articular cartilage and the osseous epiphysis. Changes may include the formation of cartilaginous flaps or free cartilaginous bodies (joint mice). The disease most commonly affects the upper humerus and sometimes affects the stifle, elbow, and hock joints. Larger breed dogs are most commonly affected. Causes are overnutrition, accelerated growth, hypervitaminosis D, and calcium deficiency.

Enostosis (eosinophilic panosteitis) is another disease of bone causing lameness and pain. Its likely cause is overnutrition.

Elbow dysplasia develops in some dogs. Parts of a bone in the elbow fail to unite with others during development and growth.

In canine wobbler syndrome the spinal canal is unable to expand during growth because normal bone remodeling in the cervical spine fails and vertebrae do not develop normally; the vertebral canal narrows, and nerve function is impaired. Overnutrition during growth is the cause.

Many degenerative diseases of bones and joints have a common basis. Undoubtedly, dogs inherit a tendency to develop these diseases. There is another important factor, however. Nutrition, particularly excesses of energy, specific vitamins, minerals, and to some extent proteins, affects bone development in many ways that are mostly detrimental. Nutrition affects the development of hip dysplasia and can lead to the above-mentioned problems, problems that proper feeding can control.

■ How Overnutrition Causes Bone and Joint Diseases

Hip dysplasia is a disease of development; puppies are not necessarily born with the problem. The problem develops during rapid growth in larger size animals. Containing growth rate reduces both the problem's frequency and severity. Unfortunately, the quality of a larger size dog is often judged by its size, with the largest size ideal. People believe that dogs achieve this ideal size through overfeeding for maximum growth. However, that is incompatible with the development of optimal skeletal growth. Moreover, nutrition alone does not decide the final size of an adult dog. Underfed puppies eventually grow to the same size as those overfed.

Overfeeding causes puppies to be overweight and has little effect on skeletal size, bone length, and diameter. People often judge a puppy's eventual size by the size of its paws. Overfeeding after weaning does not affect paw size.

Studies on overfeeding to promote weight gain in German shepherd puppies during the first two months of life showed an increased incidence of hip dysplasia at a later age. In another study, scientists compared hand-reared puppies delivered by cesarean section with puppies raised by their nursing mother. The latter puppies had hip dysplasia more frequently and with greater severity than the bottle-fed puppies. The difference was due to nursing providing more food. The first six to eight months of development are most critical for development of hip dysplasia. Feeding to support normal weight gain rather than to support maximum weight gain is essential to maintaining a low incidence of hip dysplasia.

Overfeeding to promote rapid growth prematurely stops some skeletal development. During normal growth and development, bones continue to grow and mature even after it appears that body size no longer increases. Overfeeding puppies retards bone development so that the coxafemoral acetabulum stops growing several months earlier than in puppies on a calorie-restricted diet. Overfeeding has similar effects on skeletal development in many other animals. Restricted food intake should reduce other developmental bone and joint problems in rapidly growing dogs. Unfortunately, little can be done to resolve these problems after they appear, making prevention important.

■ Diets Promoting Overfeeding

Studies on overfeeding and hip dysplasia were done with puppies eating a commercially prepared food, formulated to support growth. These diets usually contain more than the National Research Council's (NRC) recommendations for metabolizable energy, calcium, phosphorus, and protein for a growing puppy. Pet food manufacturers use the NRC recommendations and add a "fudge factor" to increase nutrients 25 percent. This permits formulation of a complete and balanced diet without its being tested in a feeding study. Puppies overeat when fed such foods free-choice, especially because they are formulated to have optimum palatability. Puppies eat more than is needed to satisfy growth and caloric needs, and many orthopedic problems develop.

Restricting their food consumption so that 17 percent less of the commercial growth diet is consumed reduces degenerative skeletal diseases. Although growth in such puppies could be retarded, a 17 percent restriction does not affect eventual body size at eight to nine months, however. More rapid growth of puppies after weaning does not translate into larger dogs at maturity.

Excessive weight gain is almost entirely due to consumption of excess calories. Dog food supplies calories primarily in the forms of carbohydrate and fat. Carbohydrate minimally promotes hip dysplasia unless carbohydrate consumption is so great that weight gain exceeds the ideal. When either dietary carbohydrate or fat contributes excess calories, orthopedic problems are more likely. Excess calories are fed more easily with fat than with carbohydrate. Puppies consume more calories with high-fat diets than with cereal-based low-fat diets because high-fat diets are more palatable. A fat-based diet containing the same number of calories as a carbohydrate-based diet is smaller volume and contributes less to satiety. Also, dietary fats burn fewer calories for conversion to a pound of adipose tissue than does the same amount of carbohydrate.

Studies report that high-protein diets do and do not promote orthopedic problems. Animal-proteins are usually high in fat, and it is likely that feeding meat results in consumption of excess calories, something that has nothing to do with meat's protein content. Puppy foods have more than adequate protein for supporting normal growth. Any excess protein will not stimulate faster growth of muscle or skeletal structures. The excess is burned for energy or converted to fat. Excess protein converted to fat results in weight gain just as excess carbohydrate converted to fat.

Vitamin C and Orthopedic Problems[3]

Vitamin C may reduce hip dysplasia and possibly other orthopedic problems. Vitamin C is involved in collagen formation, the most important structural protein. This protein found in bone and ligament makes up 25 to 30 percent of all protein. An old study reported prevention of hip dysplasias by megadoses of vitamin C given to mothers during pregnancy and after birth to puppies until young adulthood. The study involved eight litters of German shepherd puppies from parents with a history of producing puppies with hip dysplasia. The mothers received two to four grams of vitamin C per day during pregnancy. The puppies received calcium and vitamin supplements from birth to three weeks, 500 milligrams of vitamin C per day from three weeks to four months, and one to two grams of vitamin C from four months up to two years. None of the offspring had hip dysplasia. Unfortunately, no studies have been done since to confirm these results or to understand better this effect of vitamin C on hip dysplasia.

Excess vitamin C is believed to have little or no effect on the skeleton. However, excess vitamin C affects ongoing bone mineralization and resorption. Excess vitamin C increases blood calcium that is likely to delay cartilage development and maturation and interfere with bone resorption. Both affect normal bone remodeling that occurs with growth. Thus, pet foods should not contain excess vitamin C.

Hip dysplasia can develop with a degenerative disease in other joints. There is some evidence that the basis for this is increased joint laxity. Vitamin C might be necessary to prevent joint laxity; no one has proven that, however. A recent study showed that signs of chronic inflammatory joint disease (not restricted to hip dysplasia) improved when treated with vitamin C. No studies have been done to evaluate management of hip dysplasia with vitamin C.

Mineral Imbalances and Orthopedic Problems[1-3]

Many believe that rapidly growing puppies of the large to giant breed dogs have a greater than usual requirement for calcium to sustain the growth of their large skeletal structures. Consequently, they believe strongly in supplementing these puppies' diets with vitamin-mineral preparations. The fear is that not giving supplements will cause the animals to develop rickets and osteopenia.

Rickets is a disease of young growing animals that causes defective calcification of growing bone. Poorly mineralized bone deforms, giving the classical picture of rickets. Osteopenia is also a bone calcium deficiency, but it affects adults. The cause is excess diversion of calcium during pregnancy and lactation. Rickets can be due to a dietary deficiency of calcium, phosphorus, or vitamin D. Humans have rickets from vitamin D deficiency caused by inadequate exposure to sunlight. Rickets is rarely seen in dogs, and for the cases that have been observed, they are never caused by inadequate sunlight.

■ Calcium Absorption and Excretion

Excess dietary calcium does not necessarily mean that excess amounts are absorbed. Calcium absorption is determined by dietary levels of vitamin D. The liver and kidneys convert vitamin D to a derivative that stimulates intestinal calcium absorption. Calcium regulation also involves calcium's renal excretion. Thus, calcium and vitamin D supplements increase both calcium absorption and deposition. Bone calcium deposition and reabsorption are continuous processes. Their rate is at least 100 times greater in young growing animals than in adults. With a rate this high, abnormal bone growth happens more easily in young animals than adults.

■ Calcium Supplements and Orthopedic Problems

Is there any harm in oversupplementing a growing puppy with a vitamin-mineral mixture? Long-term high-calcium intake in large breed puppies can increase blood calcium and phosphate, retard bone maturation, retard bone remodeling, retard cartilage maturation, and disturb growth plates. Their manifestations include osteochondrosis, bowed legs, and stunted growth. Young dogs have no mechanisms to protect against excess dietary calcium. Excess calcium deposits primarily in bone, and with little reabsorption of bone calcium, severe abnormalities develop in the young, growing skeleton. The normal remodeling process cannot compensate for these changes.

Calcium is the major factor for skeletal disease in giant breed growing dogs. Excess dietary level of calcium is the cause. Once, rather than the level of calcium, many believed that an imbalance in the ratio of calcium to phosphorous was most important. Most nutritional recommendations over the years emphasized the need for a proper ratio of the two minerals or skeletal disease would develop. Most blamed orthopedic problems on an improper ratio.

Imbalances in the ratio of calcium to phosphorus occur most commonly when dogs eat all-meat diets. These diets often contain no bone. They are very high in phosphorus and low in calcium. The calcium to phosphorus ratio for an all-meat diet is likely to be 1:10 to 1:50. The proper ratio should be 1.3:1, or close to 1. Feeding a high-phosphorus and low-calcium diet causes calcium removal from bones to maintain normal blood calcium. Bone calcium loss results in soft bones that fracture easily.

The puppy of a giant breed is more likely than that of other breeds to show skeletal abnormalities when consuming excess calcium. This doesn't mean that excess calcium is harmless to smaller dogs. Excess calcium should not be fed to any breed of animal.

Pregnant animals often receive excess calcium. No pregnant animal, whatever its size or breed, should receive excess calcium. Feeding high levels of calcium can produce osteochondrosis in the fetus. Supplementation of calcium (but not in excess) is necessary to prevent osteopenia during pregnancy and lactation. The amount given can increase if necessary during lactation.

■ Dietary Salt and Orthopedic Problems[3]

Dietary salt concentration may be a factor in the development of hip dysplasia. Some studies show that adding an excess of salts, such as sodium and potassium, compared with others, such as chloride, to a pet's diet results in increased coxafemoral laxity, which leads to hip dysplasia.

Feeding the Large and Giant Breed Dog

Scientists do not agree on how much to feed a larger size puppy. Although criteria for deciding the caloric content of a diet for the puppy that will mature to a large or giant size are generally lacking or scanty, one can estimate the amount of energy to feed. Table 4.2 in Chapter 4 gives the caloric requirements for growing dogs that will mature to all different sizes. These values should be used as guidelines.

■ Diets for Feeding Large Breed Growing Dogs

The following diets meet a growing dog's requirements for all nutrients. They contain no more than the National Research Council's requirements for content of fats, vitamin D, calcium, and phosphorus. Feeding these diets to large breed growing dogs will make it easier to prevent the rapid growth and weight gain that lead to orthopedic problems. The diets can be supplemented with 500 milligrams of vitamin C. Vitamin B_{12} should be given by tablet several times a month or by feeding a food such as sardines that contains abundant amounts.

Chicken and Rice Diet

½ pound chicken breast meat (raw weight), cooked

2 cups rice, long-grain, cooked

1 teaspoon vegetable (canola) oil

⅓ teaspoon salt substitute—potassium chloride

¹⁄₁₀ teaspoon table salt

4 bonemeal tablets (10-grain or equivalent)

½ calcium carbonate tablet (200 milligrams calcium)

1 multiple vitamin-mineral tablet

Provides 669 kilocalories, 49.7 grams protein, 10.1 grams fat

See Table 4.2 in Chapter 4 for a puppy's caloric needs; caloric needs can be reduced up to 15 percent to minimize orthopedic problems.

Chicken and Potato Diet

½ pound chicken breast meat (raw weight), cooked

3 cups potato, cooked with skin

1 teaspoon vegetable (canola) oil

¹⁄₁₀ teaspoon table salt

4 bonemeal tablets (10-grain or equivalent)

½ calcium carbonate tablet (200 milligrams calcium)

1 multiple vitamin-mineral tablet

Provides 665 kilocalories, 49.9 grams protein, 9.7 grams fat

See Table 4.2 in Chapter 4 for a puppy's caloric needs; caloric needs can be reduced up to 15 percent to minimize orthopedic problems.

Chicken and Macaroni Diet

½ pound chicken breast meat (raw weight), cooked

2 cups macaroni, cooked

1 teaspoon vegetable (canola) oil

¼ teaspoon salt substitute—potassium chloride

¹⁄₁₀ teaspoon table salt

4 bonemeal tablets (10-grain or equivalent)

½ calcium carbonate tablet (200 milligrams calcium)

1 multiple vitamin-mineral tablet

Provides 653 kilocalories, 54.5 grams protein, 11 grams fat
See Table 4.2 in Chapter 4 for a puppy's caloric needs; caloric needs can be reduced up to 15 percent to minimize orthopedic problems.

Cottage Cheese and Rice Diet

1½ cups cottage cheese, 2 percent fat

2 cups rice, long-grain, cooked

1 teaspoon vegetable (canola) oil

¼ teaspoon salt substitute—potassium chloride

2 bonemeal tablets (10-grain or equivalent)

1 calcium carbonate tablet (400 milligrams calcium)

1 multiple vitamin-mineral tablet

Provides 760 kilocalories, 55 grams protein, 12.4 grams fat
See Table 4.2 in Chapter 4 for a puppy's caloric needs; caloric needs can be reduced up to 15 percent to minimize orthopedic problems.

Cottage Cheese and Potato Diet

1½ cups cottage cheese, 2 percent fat

3 cups potato, cooked with skin

1 teaspoon vegetable (canola) oil

2 bonemeal tablets (10-grain or equivalent)

1½ calcium carbonate tablets (600 milligrams calcium)

1 multiple vitamin-mineral tablet

Provides 756 kilocalories, 55.3 grams protein, 12 grams fat
See Table 4.2 in Chapter 4 for a puppy's caloric needs; caloric needs can be reduced up to 15 percent to minimize orthopedic problems.

Cottage Cheese and Macaroni Diet

1½ cups cottage cheese, 2 percent fat

2 cups macaroni, cooked

1 teaspoon vegetable (canola) oil

¼ teaspoon salt substitute—potassium chloride

2 bonemeal tablets (10-grain or equivalent)

1½ calcium carbonate tablets (600 milligrams calcium)

1 multiple vitamin-mineral tablet

Provides 744 kilocalories, 60 grams protein, 13.4 grams fat
See Table 4.2 in Chapter 4 for a puppy's caloric needs; caloric needs can be reduced up to 15 percent to minimize orthopedic problems.

Information on overnutrition causing orthopedic problems is recent. During the last 50 years veterinarians were usually happy to see owners bring in well-fed puppies of any breed. An owner was usually instructed and encouraged to feed a puppy so it looked as healthy as possible. "Healthy" most importantly meant that it was not thin. Now it is known that this approach is wrong, especially if the puppy will mature to a large size. If a puppy is fed so that the owner can be proud of its size, orthopedic problems can be expected.

Management of Osteoarthritis

Osteoarthritis is one of the most common ailments of both young and old dogs: it is also a problem in some cats. The problem is helped by reducing weight in obese animals. Osteoarthritis is treated most often with nonsteroidal antiinflammatory drugs and sometimes with surgery. Drug treatment must be continuous, and results are often unsatisfactory. These drugs cause serious side effects by inhibiting prostaglandin production. When its levels are reduced, the gastrointestinal mucosa ulcerates. This effect is so severe that many will not use nonsteroidal inflammatory drugs in dogs.

Newer management of osteoarthritis includes dietary supplementation with forms of cartilage. This treatment has not found favor with clinicians, but there have been no controlled studies to show that giving cartilage doesn't help. Dogs with moderate osteoarthritis causing clinical signs of lameness for four to five months have improved dramatically with cartilage supplementation. (No comparable trials have been done on cats.) Cartilage can be given in the form of a commercially prepared supplement, with an 80-pound dog receiving *three* 750-milligram tablets *daily* or *three* tablets *daily* containing a combination of chondroitin (400 mg) and glucosamine (500 mg). If a dog is fed chicken, the cartilage on the ends of bones can be easily removed after boiling and included in the meal.[4]

It is not known why cartilage benefits animals with osteoarthritis. Some believe that glycosaminoglycans released from digested cartilage are absorbed and enter joints, where they help renew damaged articular surfaces. Cartilage given orally also inhibits intestinal absorption of toxins, and that could benefit arthritis. Some cases of arthritis are associated with chronic inflammatory bowel disease, and the arthritis is suspected to result from toxic substances absorbed from the intestine. Cartilage is poorly digested so that no more than half is degraded. Cartilage is a complex carbohydrate that binds both bacterial toxins in the intestine and the intestine's mucosal surface. Both of these actions reduce toxin absorption.

Because some animals can benefit from cartilage and the product is safe and relatively inexpensive, the first attempt in managing osteoarthritis should be to give cartilage. Patients given cartilage and responding to it have shown little or no lameness after three weeks.

Summary

In summary, many factors are involved in the development of hip dysplasia and other orthopedic problems. It is difficult to control factors such as breed predisposition other than by not breeding affected animals. That has not solved the problems. Other factors can be controlled. Maximum growth rate should be prevented. Growth rate can be controlled by restricting caloric intake 15 to 20 percent of usual recommendations; excess weight gain has been linked to the development of hip dysplasia. Restriction of caloric intake during growth has no effect on eventual size at maturity. Such restriction does determine normal skeletal integrity during and after growth.

Deficiencies of specific nutrients are rare and should not be such a concern that an excess of any nutrient is fed. Excess calcium and vitamin D cause orthopedic problems from the absorption of excess calcium. Excess nutrients are not harmless because the animal cannot compensate for the excess of many. Large dogs may be less able to compensate than smaller animals. Rickets and other deficiency diseases are rare today.

Many believe that canine orthopedic problems are largely caused by genetic defects, and culling of carriers has been proposed. These problems were infrequent more than 50 years ago, at a time when not many dogs ate commercial pet foods. Many of these orthopedic problems are genetic problems, but they manifest because of overnutrition.

Owners are forced to feed puppies free-choice because they lack useful information to do otherwise. Pet food labels provide vague information on the proper amount to feed a puppy. As a result, owners give puppies as much food as they want. Instead of feeding puppies to look well fed and to achieve a size to be proud of, they should be fed amounts that allow them to appear lean and trim.

Animals with osteoarthritis should be managed by weight reduction, where indicated, and by cartilage given orally.

References

1. Hazewinkel, Herman A.W. 1994. Skeletal disease. In *The Waltham Book of Clinical Nutrition of the Dog and Cat*, edited by J.M. Wills and K.W. Simpson, 395–423. Oxford: Pergamon Press.

2. Kealy, Richard D., Dennis Frank Lawler, Joan Marion Ballam, George Lust, Gail Keen Smith, Daryl Norman Biery, and Sten Eric Olsson. 1997. Five-

year longitudinal study on limited food consumption and development of osteoarthritis in coxofemoral joints of dogs. *Journal of the American Veterinary Medical Association* 210(2):222–225.

3. Richardson, Daniel C. 1992. The role of nutrition in canine hip dsyplasia. *Veterinary Clinics of North America: Small Animal Practice* 22(3):529–540.

4. Altman, R.D., D.D. Dean, and O.E. Muniz et al. 1989. Therapeutic treatment of canine osteoarthritis with glycosaminoglycan polysulfuric acid ester. *Arthritis and Rheumatism* 32:1300–1307.

PART FIVE
Dietary Management of Disease

CHAPTER 13
Diet and Chronic Renal Disease

Renal disease affects an unusually large number of dogs and cats. It affects 1 percent of all age dogs and at least 10 percent of dogs over 15 years old. These estimates are probably low. Most likely the incidence is similar for cats. Although chronic renal disease is easily identified, moderate damage is probably more common and not recognized because signs do not appear until renal damage is severe.

Early recognition and management of renal disease are important for two reasons. Renal damage is irreversible; animals lose structure and function in affected nephrons. Second, renal damage is progressive, so if untreated, normal nephrons are destroyed. Management's goal is to preserve normal nephrons. With progressive damage, animal mortality is high, and treatment is costly; dialysis and renal transplantation are often necessary.

Feeding affected animals a controlled diet usually preserves remaining nephron function. Diets must have proper amounts of calcium, magnesium, sodium, and potassium, and often they must be formulated with reduced phosphorus. Concentrations of some vitamins must not exceed requirements. Dietary protein is sometimes reduced to a minimum. Some studies show benefits from reducing protein consumption, but other studies show no benefits. The nature of a renal problem determines dietary protein levels.

Understanding how renal disease is developed is important to its dietary management. A knowledge of causes for renal damage also helps to determine how dietary management can prevent chronic renal disease.

Etiology

■ Acute Disease[1-3]

Renal disease develops following many acute insults. Acute disease is often caused by nephrotoxins. Common toxins include antibiotics such as aminoglycosides and amphotericin B, antifreeze (ethylene glycol), and nonsteroidal antiinflammatory drugs.

An important cause of acute renal damage is excess vitamin D. Commonly used rodenticides contain vitamin D. When ingested, they promote excess calcium absorption. Excess calcium crystallizing in renal tissue destroys nephrons. Poisoning with vitamin D kills by acute renal failure.

Acute renal damage also develops when renal blood flow is severely reduced. Additional causes include chronic renal infection or inflammation and disease in other organs.

■ Chronic Disease[1,2]

Renal disease is not usually identified until it is chronic, probably because most owners do not recognize clinical signs of early disease. Many different causes have been suggested to be the most significant. Fifty years ago, the most important cause was thought to be leptospirosis infection. Now this disease is rare, and other explanations are necessary for the causes of renal disease. The causes can be similar to those for acute problems. But these causes cannot explain the high incidence of chronic renal disease.

Toxins infrequently cause chronic renal damage, and chronic infectious disease or inflammatory disease can infrequently be targeted as the cause of chronic renal disease either. With these secondary causes, management to correct the primary problem should cause renal damage to stop and renal function to stabilize.

What best explains the high incidence of kidney disease in dogs and cats? Dogs and cats should not be so unique that they have chronic renal disease much more commonly than other mammals, including humans. This frequency may relate to feeding commercial pet foods; the rate has been increasing with their feeding. Commercial foods can cause problems when they contain excess vitamin D; earlier it was noted that this vitamin is indirectly a nephrotoxin.

Vitamin D is added to pet foods during processing, and manufacturers do not measure its amount in the finished product. As with most vitamins, D is added in excess to ensure that an adequate amount remains after the predicted loss during cooking. Manufacturers believe vitamins are safe so that addition of larger amounts should be of little consequence. However, addition of excess vitamins to commerical pet foods can be important in causing medical problems.

The imprecise addition of vitamin D to milk processed for human consumption has caused vitamin D toxicity that resulted in some human deaths. Could that happen from pet foods? It is not likely that large amounts of vitamin D would be added and result in acute toxicity, such as with a rodent poison. But it is possible that "excess but safe" amounts added to pet foods result in subclinical toxicity. Over a period of months or years, that excess could eventually damage the kidneys so that they fail, resulting in signs of disease. An unusually high incidence of chronic renal disease in cats has been associated with a brand of cat food containing high levels of vitamin D.

Excessive dietary levels of calcium and phosphorus can also lead to mineralization in the kidneys of normal animals. Diets should contain proper amounts of these minerals.

Pathogenesis of Renal Damage[1,4,5]

■ Calcium and Phosphorus

Calcium is present in animal tissues as a free (soluble) and a bound form. The concentration of free intracellular calcium is very low, thousands of times lower than extracellular concentration of calcium. Increased free intracellular calcium damages and kills cells and is the most important reason for cell injury and death due to any cause. Anything increasing intracellular free calcium levels damages cells. Increased extracellular calcium or phosphorus can increase intracellular free calcium concentration.

Abnormal extracellular calcium and phosphorus concentration also causes calcium and phosphate crystallization in nephrons. Crystals cause inflammation, scarring, and nephron loss.

Many different diseases can increase extracellular calcium and phosphorus levels to cause renal damage and failure. Causes of high extracellular calcium include lymphoma and parathyroid gland tumors that secrete excess parathormone or parathormone-like substances. Excess dietary calcium or vitamin D also increases extracellular calcium. Excess dietary phosphorus, a low dietary calcium-to-phosphorus ratio, low magnesium intake, and renal disease resulting in a failure of phosphorus excretion are all causes of renal calcium and phosphate crystallization.

■ Vitamin D Excess

Vitamin D is necessary for dietary calcium and phosphorus absorption. Deficiency of vitamin D was one of the common causes of calcium and phosphorus deficiency (rickets) in dogs some years ago. Excess vitamin D promotes absorption of excess dietary calcium and phosphorus. Excess dietary vitamin D is toxic and has the potential for being the most toxic vitamin. Toxic levels promote deposition of calcium and phosphate as crystals in the kidneys, heart, and major blood vessels.

■ Hypertension

High blood pressure is relatively uncommon in dogs and cats compared with humans. Chronic renal disease is the most common cause for high blood pressure in dogs and cats. Hypertension may be the most critical factor causing progression of renal damage.

Chronically diseased kidneys have fewer nephrons, and these are overworked, something that contributes to ongoing nephron destruction. Hypertension results from the increased renal blood flow needed to sustain the increased workload for remaining nephrons. Management is directed at minimizing the renal workload. One primary renal burden is excretion of waste products resulting from protein metabolism. A restricted-protein diet is fed to manage this burden. Hypertension, and the damage it causes, is managed by restricting sodium intake. Drugs should not replace dietary management to correct hypertension.

■ Acidosis and Ammonia

The kidneys play an important role in maintaining acid-base homeostasis. Dietary protein is metabolized to acid products that the kidneys must excrete. These acid products result primarily from the metabolism of sulfur-containing amino acids and phosphates. Renal excretion of acid produces ammonia, which is toxic to kidney cells. Renal ammonia formation can be reduced by feeding a diet that minimizes acid.

Sulfur-containing amino acids and phosphates are highest in animal proteins. Plant proteins are low in sulfur amino acids and high in salts and minerals such as potassium and magnesium, which promote alkaline rather than acid conditions. The acid effects of a diet can be reduced by giving an alkalinizing agent such as sodium bicarbonate, potassium citrate, or calcium carbonate.

■ Lipids

Abnormal lipid metabolism is found in humans and sometimes in animals with renal disease. Abnormalities may result from renal disease, and some may contribute to its progression. Abnormal changes include hyperlipidemia and possibly hypercholesterolemia. Management can include reducing dietary cholesterol and saturated fats. Some benefit may be gained by feeding more polyunsaturated fat.

Diagnosis[1,2]

There are no specific signs alerting owners to renal disease. Nonspecific signs such as increased water consumption, loss of appetite, vomiting, depression, and weight loss are common. However, these signs are not specific for renal disease. Early signs should not be ignored because more significant signs do not appear until most renal function is lost. The loss is irreversible.

Renal disease is diagnosed by laboratory tests that include a urinalysis and blood chemistries. The urinalysis is helpful in evaluating the kidney functions of diluting and concentrating urine. It also helps identify infection and active inflammation. However, a urinalysis can have normal results if renal disease is present, so an evaluation must include additional tests.

Blood chemistry tests evaluate blood urea and often creatinine, both of which increase with chronic renal disease. Blood chemistry tests also evaluate plasma phosphorus and calcium, which can increase with reduced renal function. Potassium is also excreted renally, and its blood levels can increase with reduced renal function. (With vomiting and inappetence potassium losses can be excessive, resulting in hypokalemia.) When renal disease reduces excretion of acid products, acidosis develops and appears on blood chemistry evaluations as reduced bicarbonate concentration.

A complete blood count identifies anemia, an important complication of chronic renal disease. The kidney produces erythropoietin, which is necessary for bone marrow to produce erythrocytes.

Erythropoietin production may be deficient with renal disease. Erythropoietin is used to treat anemia due to chronic renal disease.

Blood pressure is measured to identify hypertension. Dietary management changes with hypertension.

Other tests to evaluate for chronic renal disease are not essential. A renal biopsy gives information on the extent of damage and is usually done for prognosis. No other tests contribute additional new and useful information for evaluating most animals with chronic renal disease.

Feeding to Restrict Renal Damage[1,2,6,7]

■ Dietary Protein Selection and Restriction

Dietary protein should be restricted for some dogs and cats with chronic renal disease. That restriction reduces the exposure of nephrons to toxins and reduces their work. As noted above, some products of protein metabolism are toxic, so feeding a low-protein diet reduces toxin damage. Reducing dietary protein also decreases renal excretion of waste products. Reduced protein diets limit (1) proteinuria, (2) glomerular damage, and (3) progressive loss of renal function.

Protein restriction generally reduces phosphorus intake. Mostly meat diets are rich in phosphorus, and some years ago they caused many problems until manufacturers balanced them by adding calcium. Phosphorus is toxic, as already described. It causes calcium phosphate crystallization, which damages nephrons. In all of the following diets, phosphorus levels are low to very low, and that reflects not the protein source as much as the protein amount.

The optimal value of a restricted-protein diet is most importantly determined by feeding proteins with high biological value. Little of these proteins is catabolized to products (urea, phosphate, and sulfate) the kidneys must excrete. Egg protein has the highest biological value (set at 100) and so is ideal for dietary management of chronic renal disease. For comparison, the biological value for milk protein is 92, chicken or beef 78, soybean protein (tofu) 73, oat protein 65, rice protein 64, and corn protein 45.[8]

Egg protein is high in sulfur-containing amino acids, however, but unless acidosis is marked (usually only in severe or terminal cases), eggs are the ideal protein to feed. On the other hand, sulfur-containing amino acids are the first limiting amino acids in milk and soybean proteins. This means that relative to the other essential amino acids they provide the smallest percentage of an animal's requirement.

Diets with proteins from vegetables rather than animals are low in sulfur-containing amino acids and produce less acid. However, because the biological value for vegetable protein is much lower than that for animal protein, more protein must be consumed, and that increases waste for renal excretion. Thus, with the possible exception of tofu, the protein in the following diets is from animals.

Affected dogs require two to three and one-half grams of protein per kilogram of body weight per day. The lower amount can be used when feeding a protein with a high biological value, and the higher amount when feeding a protein with low biological value. Feeding a low–biological value protein requires more work from kidneys with reduced function. Feeding a diet containing a high-quality protein such as casein maintains an adult dog at a protein level of 6.5 percent of the diet's dry matter. In general, feeding high-quality protein diets containing 8 to 10 percent protein maintains adult dogs.

The amount of protein to feed cats with kidney disease is 24 percent crude protein (minimum requirement for an adult cat: three and one-half grams per kilogram of body weight); the protein must have a high biological value. The diet must provide a proper balance between the amounts of crude protein and calories. For maintenance of healthy adult cats, the ratio of grams of protein to megacalories of energy should be at least 65 (65 grams of protein for each 1000 kilocalories fed). In cats with chronic kidney disease, reduce this ratio to 55 during the early stages of disease and to about 45 as the severity of kidney failure progresses.

■ Dietary Phosphate Restriction

Dietary phosphorus is reduced in proportion to renal impairment. The primary biochemical abnormalities with loss of renal function are uremia and azotemia. These changes are not usually evident until renal functional capacity is reduced to 25 percent or less. Based on this, dietary phosphorus intake should be decreased to 25 percent of normal.

The National Research Council (NRC) recommends that normal dogs receive 89 milligrams phosphorus per kilogram body weight per day. There is little information from studies on cats to show how much phosphorus a normal adult should receive. The level of phosphorus is about 1.3 percent in commercial pet foods. Dogs with chronic kidney disease and azotemia will develop hyperphosphatemia with this dietary level of phosphorus. Nutritionists recommend a low dietary level of phosphorus, about 0.35 percent for both dogs and cats with chronic renal disease. Whatever the level, it must be low enough to prevent hyperphosphatemia.

The dietary ratio of calcium to phosphorus should be greater than 1; an even higher ratio may be beneficial. Calcium can be supplemented, except when blood calcium is increased.

Blood phosphorus levels can be reduced by phosphorus binders given orally. Calcium carbonate binds phosphorus and can be used unless blood calcium is high. Other binders include phytin found in vegetable matter and antacid salts of magnesium or aluminum. Magnesium can help correct a low magnesium-to-phosphorus ratio, but it can also result in hypermagnesemia, which must be avoided. In the following diets phosphorus is low enough that binding agents are unnecessary.

In summary, to restrict phosphorus, feed a diet that is low in phosphorus and has the proper ratio of phosphorus to calcium. If more severe restriction requires some of the other measures, renal disease is so critical that it is not likely to respond well.

■ Dietary Salt Restriction—Controlling Hypertension

Hypertension of renal circulation may be the critical determinant of renal disease progressing. As noted earlier, protein restriction relieves hypertension because renal blood flow lessens. This hypertension can be managed by two other means, both being dietary.

Reduction of dietary sodium is essential for normalizing blood pressure. Commercial dog foods are high-salt diets. Manufacturers include up to 1 percent sodium chloride in dry dog foods, which provides approximately 95 milligrams sodium and 147 milligrams chloride per kilogram of body weight per day. With kidney disease sodium is restricted to 15–50 milligrams sodium per kilogram of body weight daily. If necessary, sodium intake is restricted to the NRC recommended minimum daily requirement of 11 milligrams sodium per kilogram of body weight.

No minimum requirement is established for sodium or salt in cats. Cats tolerate diets containing 1 percent salt, but that level is excessive. A level of 0.24 percent salt may be necessary for managing cats with chronic renal disease.

Reduction of hypertension is also possible with weight reduction in obese dogs. A relationship has been established between obesity and hypertension in dogs.

Medications can be used to manage hypertension. They may be necessary with severe renal disease; until then hypertension should be managed dietarily.

■ Dietary Potassium Restriction or Supplementation

Chronic renal disease greatly increases urine production in some dogs. Such animals can lose large amounts of potassium and become deficient. Potassium depletion can be difficult to identify because blood potassium can be either normal or low. Commercial dry dog foods contain from 0.70 to 0.85 percent potassium. The NRC recommends a dietary level of 0.44 percent potassium. Hypokalemic animals should be given 1 to 6 mEq (about 40 to 235 milligrams) potassium per kilogram body weight per day.

Cats are more likely to develop hypokalemia than dogs. Cats require supplementation with potassium to a dietary level of at least 0.5 to 0.6 percent. (The minimum dietary recommendation by the NRC is 0.4 percent.) Because sodium reduces potassium levels, the dietary ratio of potassium to sodium is maintained at 2 to 1 or greater. Acidosis complicating chronic renal disease can worsen hypokalemia. Drugs for acidifying urine can also cause acidosis.

Because hyperkalemia is serious and life threatening, potassium intake must be reduced. Specific treatment for hyperkalemia involves intravenous glucose (with or without insulin) or bicarbonate solutions.

■ Dietary Magnesium Intake

Urinary tract struvite stones form in cats for a number of interrelated reasons. Diets containing greater than 0.35 percent magnesium were once related to stone formation. In response manufacturers formulated cat foods with little magnesium. This resulted in hypomagnesemia, which increases urinary potassium excretion and leads to hypokalemia. Adequate amounts of magnesium are also needed to prevent calcium crystallization and renal stone formation. For cats, dietary magnesium should be 0.10 to 0.12 percent, compared with the NRC recommended minimum level of 0.04 percent. Canine requirements are satisfied with a dietary level of 0.05 percent magnesium.

■ Dietary Energy Intake

Animals with renal disease are fed to maintain normal body weight. If necessary, caloric intake is adjusted so underweight dogs regain weight losses and overweight dogs lose weight. Restricting caloric intake to minimum basic needs may be beneficial for slowing the progression of chronic renal disease.

■ Dietary Lipid Selection and Restriction

Reducing dietary saturated fat and cholesterol may benefit dogs with chronic renal disease. Nonanimal protein is needed for that. (However, it is far more important to select proteins of animal origin in order to feed those with the highest biologic value.) In addition, foods rich in polyunsaturated fatty acids such as fish or vegetable oil are fed to meet unsaturated fatty acid and caloric needs. These fatty acids relieve hypercholesterolemia and hyperlipidemia in some dogs with chronic renal disease. Some experimental studies suggest that polyunsaturated fatty acids may adversely affect renal function in chronic renal disease. Polyunsaturated fatty acids are precursors for leukotrienes and prostaglandins. High dietary levels may promote formation of inflammatory mediators and thereby worsen renal damage. That is unproven, however, and substituting polyunsaturated fatty acids that produce mediators with weaker inflammatory properties (omega-3 polyunsaturated fatty acids) does not benefit animals with renal disease.

Dietary fats are important for other reasons. Low-fat diets are unpalatable, and anorexic cats with chronic renal disease are unlikely to eat any low-fat diet. These cats also suffer from weight loss, and feeding to promote weight gain must include more than minimal amounts of fats. The dietary fat content on a dry basis should be at least 13 to 15 percent. Vegetable and fish oils are selected unless others, such as chicken fat, offering better palatability, are available.

■ Vitamin and Trace Mineral Supplementation

Chronic renal disease is associated with reduced intestinal absorption and increased urinary losses of some trace minerals. Iron and zinc deficiencies are possible, and supplements of these elements should be given. Iron is necessary for erythrocyte production, and with chronic renal disease often causing anemia, additional iron may benefit some.

Vitamin deficiencies are also likely because of reduced intestinal absorption and increased urinary losses. Diets are supplemented with B complex vitamins, vitamin C, and vitamin K. It is dangerous to give additional vitamin D. Commercial pet foods may contain excess vitamin D, which can be responsible for chronic renal disease. As mentioned earlier vitamin D promotes calcium absorption, and high intracellular calcium damages renal cells. Protection of the remaining nephrons against further damage is accomplished by minimizing dietary vitamin D.

Diets for Management of Chronic Renal Disease in Dogs

The following diets supply nutrients for a medium size adult dog and provide about 10 percent protein (135 percent of needs). Chicken fat improves palatability. Increasing dietary chicken fat decreases the protein percent, however. The diets are all low in phosphorus and provide 50 to 75 percent of vitamin D requirements. Some diets contain minimum amounts of sodium, and some are deficient in sodium. Some animals lose excess sodium with chronic renal disease, and in such cases iodized salt is used for flavor (one-tenth teaspoon iodized salt can be added). These diets contain normal, low, or high amounts of potassium and should be fed according to the dog's needs. Potassium-depleted animals can be fed a low-potassium diet if one-fourth teaspoon potassium chloride is added. Magnesium is available to meet required levels. Some diets are low in vitamin B_{12}, which is probably unimportant unless they are fed for many months. Substituting chicken or ground beef for eggs enhances flavor and provides more B complex and B_{12} vitamins. A vitamin B_{12} supplement can be given occasionally. The diets are balanced with respect to all other nutrients.

Feeding a diet matched to needs can restore phosphorus, potassium, and sodium to normal. Blood chemistry panels are done to monitor plasma concentrations. With normal blood levels dietary mineral levels can be modified. It may not be necessary to continue feeding a very low phosphorus diet; doing so may result in a deficiency.

To increase a dog's dietary phosphorus, substitute bonemeal tablets for calcium carbonate tablets. For example, to one of these diets providing 45 percent of the phosphorus needs, adding four bonemeal tablets (10-grain tablets) in place of one and one-half calcium carbonate tablets increases the dietary phosphate to meet National Research Council requirements. Normal calcium levels are maintained. At the end of each recipe, directions are given for restoring normal phosphorus levels.

Egg and Potato Diet (*Low-protein, low-phosphorus, high-potassium, normal sodium*)

1 egg, large, cooked

3 cups potato, boiled with skin

1 tablespoon chicken fat

1½ calcium carbonate tablets (600 milligrams calcium)

½ multiple vitamin-mineral tablet

Provides 600 kilocalories, 15.1 grams protein, 18.5 grams fat
Supports caloric needs of an 18-pound dog
Provides phosphorus at 53 percent, potassium at 322 percent, sodium at 114 percent of dog's daily needs. To feed this diet with a normal amount of phosphorus, substitute 3 bone-meal tablets for the 1½ calcium carbonate tablets.

Chicken and Potato Diet (*Low-protein, low-phosphorus, high-potassium, low-sodium*)

¼ cup cooked chicken breast

3 cups potato, boiled with skin

2 tablespoons chicken fat

1½ calcium carbonate tablets (600 milligrams calcium)

½ multiple vitamin-mineral tablet

Provides 689 kilocalories, 18.9 grams protein, 26.8 grams fat
Supports caloric needs of a 21- to 22-pound dog
Provides phosphorus at 45 percent, potassium at 301 percent, sodium at 54 percent of a dog's daily needs. To feed this diet with a normal amount of phosphorus, substitute 4 bone-meal tablets for the 1½ calcium carbonate tablets.

Beef and Potato Diet (*Low-protein, low-phosphorus, high-potassium, low-sodium*)

2 ounces lean ground beef (raw weight), cooked

3 cups potato, boiled with skin

2 tablespoons chicken fat

1½ calcium carbonate tablets (600 milligrams calcium)

½ multiple vitamin-mineral tablet

Provides 737 kilocalories, 18.6 grams protein, 32.5 grams fat
Supports caloric needs of a 23- to 24-pound dog
Provides phosphorus at 43 percent, potassium at 293 percent, sodium at 54 percent of a dog's daily needs. To feed this diet with a normal amount of phosphorus, substitute 4 bonemeal tablets for the 1½ calcium carbonate tablets.

Eggs and Tapioca Diet (*Low-protein, low-phosphorus, low-potassium, normal sodium*)

3 eggs, large, hard-boiled

2 cups tapioca, cooked (125 grams dry before cooking)

1 tablespoon chicken fat

1½ calcium carbonate tablets (600 milligrams calcium)

½ multiple vitamin-mineral tablet

Provides 779 kilocalories, 19.3 grams protein, 28.9 grams fat
Supports caloric needs of a 25-pound dog
Provides phosphorus at 40 percent, potassium at 30 percent, sodium at 216 percent of a dog's daily needs. To feed this diet with a normal amount of phosphorus, substitute 4 bonemeal tablets for the 1½ calcium carbonate tablets.

Beef and Tapioca Diet *(Low-protein, low-phosphorus, low-potas-sium, low-sodium)*

4 ounces lean ground beef (raw weight), cooked

2 cups tapioca, cooked (125 grams dry before cooking)

2 tablespoons chicken fat

1½ calcium carbonate tablets (600 milligrams calcium)

½ multiple vitamin-mineral tablet

Provides 845 kilocalories, 19.9 grams protein, 37.2 grams fat
Supports caloric needs of a 28-pound dog
Provides phosphorus at 18 percent, potassium at 29 per-cent, sodium at 55 percent of a dog's daily needs. To feed this diet with a normal amount of phosphorus, substitute 5 to 6 bonemeal tablets for the 1½ calcium carbonate tablets.

Egg Whites and Tapioca Diet *(Low-protein, low-phosphorus, low-potassium, normal sodium)*

Egg whites from 3 eggs, hard-boiled

2 cups tapioca, cooked (125 grams dry before cooking)

1 tablespoon chicken fat

1½ calcium carbonate tablets (600 milligrams calcium)

½ multiple vitamin-mineral tablet

Provides 610 kilocalories, 14.1 grams protein, 13 grams fat
Supports caloric needs of an 18-pound dog
Provides phosphorus at 6 percent, potassium at 33 percent, sodium at 269 percent of a dog's daily needs. To feed this diet with a normal amount of phosphorus, substitute 6 bonemeal tablets for the 1½ calcium carbonate tablets.

Chicken and Tapioca Diet (Low-protein, low-phosphorus, low-potassium, low-sodium)

½ cup cooked chicken breast

2 cups tapioca, cooked (125 grams dry before cooking)

2 tablespoons chicken fat

1½ calcium carbonate tablets (600 milligrams calcium)

½ multiple vitamin-mineral tablet

Provides 763 kilocalories, 20.8 grams protein, 27.3 grams fat
Supports caloric needs of a 24- to 25-pound dog
Provides phosphorus at 20 percent, potassium at 22 percent, sodium at 55 percent of a dog's daily needs. To feed this diet with a normal amount of phosphorus, substitute 5 to 6 bonemeal tablets for the 1½ calcium carbonate tablets.

Eggs and Rice Diet (Low-protein, low-phosphorus, low-potassium, normal sodium)

1 egg, large, hard-boiled

2 cups rice, long-grain, cooked

1 tablespoon chicken fat

1½ calcium carbonate tablets (600 milligrams calcium)

½ multiple vitamin-mineral tablet

Provides 721 kilocalories, 15.2 grams protein, 31.4 grams fat
Supports caloric needs of a 23-pound dog
Provides phosphorus at 40 percent, potassium at 30 percent, sodium at 90 percent of a dog's daily needs. To feed this diet with a normal amount of phosphorus, substitute 4 bonemeal tablets for the 1½ calcium carbonate tablets.

Egg Whites and Rice Diet (Low-protein, low-phosphorus, low-potassium, normal sodium)

Egg whites from 3 eggs, large, hard-boiled

2 cups rice, long-grain, cooked

2 tablespoons chicken fat

1½ calcium carbonate tablets (600 milligrams calcium)

½ multiple vitamin-mineral tablet

Provides 693 kilocalories, 18.8 grams protein, 26.8 grams fat
Supports caloric needs of a 21- to 22-pound dog
Provides phosphorus at 27 percent, potassium at 43 percent, sodium at 208 percent of a dog's daily needs. To feed this diet with a normal amount of phosphorus, substitute 5 bone-meal tablets for the 1½ calcium carbonate tablets.

Diets for Management of Chronic Renal Disease in Cats

Chicken and Rice Diet (Low-protein, low-phosphorus, normal potassium, normal sodium diet providing 55 grams protein/1000 kilocalories)

¼ cup cooked chicken breast

½ ounce clams, canned, chopped in juice

½ cup rice, long-grain, cooked

1 tablespoon chicken fat

⅛ teaspoon salt substitute—potassium chloride

1 calcium carbonate tablet (400 milligrams calcium)

¼ multiple vitamin-mineral tablet

⅒ B complex vitamin–trace mineral tablet

Provides 297 kilocalories, 16.3 grams protein, 14.5 grams fat
See Table 4.4 in Chapter 4 for caloric needs of cats.
Provides phosphorus at 48 percent, potassium at 215 percent, sodium at 169 percent of a cat's daily needs. To feed this diet with a normal amount of phosphorus, substitute 3 bone-meal tablets for the 1 calcium carbonate tablet.

Chicken and Rice Diet (Low-protein, low-phosphorus, normal potassium, normal sodium diet providing 46.4 grams protein/1000 kilocalories)

¼ cup cooked chicken breast

½ ounce clams, canned, chopped in juice

1 cup rice, long-grain, cooked

1 tablespoon chicken fat

⅛ teaspoon salt substitute—potassium chloride

1 calcium carbonate tablet (400 milligrams calcium)

¼ multiple vitamin-mineral tablet

1/10 B complex vitamin–trace mineral tablet

Provides 399 kilocalories, 18.5 grams protein, 14.7 grams fat
See Table 4.4 in Chapter 4 for caloric needs of cats.

Provides phosphorus at 43 percent, potassium at 164 percent, sodium at 124 percent of a cat's daily needs. To feed this diet with a normal amount of phosphorus, substitute 3 bonemeal tablets for the 1 calcium carbonate tablet.

Egg Whites and Rice Diet (Low-protein, low-phosphorus, normal potassium, normal sodium diet providing 53 grams protein/1000 kilocalories)

Egg whites from 3 eggs, large, hard-boiled

1 ounce clams, canned, chopped in juice

½ cup rice, long-grain, cooked

1 tablespoon chicken fat

⅛ teaspoon salt substitute—potassium chloride

1½ calcium carbonate tablets (600 milligrams calcium)

¼ multiple vitamin-mineral tablet

1/10 B complex vitamin–trace mineral tablet

Provides 312 kilocalories, 19.7 grams protein, 13.8 grams fat
See Table 4.4 in Chapter 4 for caloric needs of cats.

Provides phosphorus at 41 percent, potassium at 341 percent, sodium at 603 percent of a cat's daily needs. To feed this diet with a normal amount of phosphorus, substitute 3 bone-meal tablets for the $1\frac{1}{2}$ calcium carbonate tablets.

Egg Whites and Rice Diet (Low-protein, low-phosphorus, normal potassium, normal sodium diet providing 46.6 grams protein/1000 kilocalories)

Egg whites from 2 eggs, large, hard-boiled

1 ounce clams, canned, chopped in juice

1 cup rice, long-grain, cooked

1 tablespoon chicken fat

$\frac{1}{8}$ teaspoon salt substitute—potassium chloride

$1\frac{1}{2}$ calcium carbonate tablets (600 milligrams calcium)

$\frac{1}{4}$ multiple vitamin-mineral tablet

$\frac{1}{10}$ B complex vitamin–trace mineral tablet

Provides 399 kilocalories, 18.6 grams protein, 13.9 grams fat
See Table 4.4 in Chapter 4 for caloric needs of cats.

Provides phosphorus at 41 percent, potassium at 341 percent, sodium at 603 percent of a cat's daily needs. To feed this diet with a normal amount of phosphorus, substitute 3 bone-meal tablets for the $1\frac{1}{2}$ calcium carbonate tablets.

Egg Diet (Low-protein, low-phosphorus, normal potassium, normal sodium diet providing 54.2 grams protein/1000 kilocalories)

2 eggs, large, hard-boiled

$\frac{1}{2}$ ounce clams, canned, chopped in juice

1 tablespoon chicken fat

⅛ teaspoon salt substitute—potassium chloride

1 calcium carbonate tablet (400 milligrams calcium)

¼ multiple vitamin-mineral tablet

⅒ B complex vitamin–trace mineral tablet

Provides 308 kilocalories, 16.7 grams protein, 25 grams fat
See Table 4.4 in Chapter 4 for caloric needs of cats.

Provides phosphorus at 89 percent, potassium at 274 percent, sodium at 673 percent of a cat's daily needs. Bonemeal need not be used in this diet to increase phosphorus content.

Eggs and Rice Diet (Low-protein, low-phosphorus, normal potassium, normal sodium diet providing 45.7 grams protein/1000 kilocalories)

2 eggs, large, hard-boiled

½ ounce clams, canned, chopped in juice

½ cup rice, long-grain, cooked

1 tablespoon chicken fat

⅛ teaspoon salt substitute—potassium chloride

1 calcium carbonate tablet (400 milligrams calcium)

¼ multiple vitamin-mineral tablet

⅒ B complex vitamin–trace mineral tablet

Provides 411 kilocalories, 18.8 grams protein, 25.2 grams fat
See Table 4.4 in Chapter 4 for caloric needs of cats.

Provides phosphorus at 69 percent, potassium at 189 percent, sodium at 440 percent of a cat's daily needs. To feed this diet with a normal amount of phosphorus, substitute 1 bonemeal tablet and ½ calcium carbonate tablet for 1 calcium carbonate tablet.

Chicken and Potato Diet (*Low-protein, low-phosphorus, normal potassium, normal sodium diet providing 57.4 grams protein/1000 kilocalories*)

½ cup cooked chicken breast

½ ounce clams, canned, chopped in juice

½ cup potato, boiled with skin

2 tablespoons chicken fat

1½ calcium carbonate tablets (600 milligrams calcium)

¼ multiple vitamin-mineral tablet

¹/₁₀ B complex vitamin–trace mineral tablet

Provides 453 kilocalories, 26 grams protein, 30.6 grams fat
See Table 4.4 in Chapter 4 for caloric needs of cats.
Provides phosphorus at 52 percent, potassium at 198 percent, sodium at 201 percent of daily a cat's needs. To feed this diet with a normal amount of phosphorus, substitute 3 bone-meal tablets for the 1½ calcium carbonate tablets.

Chicken and Potato Diet (*Low-protein, low-phosphorus, normal potassium, normal sodium diet providing 46.2 grams protein/1000 kilocalories*)

⅓ cup cooked chicken breast

½ ounce clams, canned, chopped in juice

½ cup potato, boiled with skin

2 tablespoons chicken fat

1½ calcium carbonate tablets (600 milligrams calcium)

¹/₄ multiple vitamin-mineral tablet

¹/₁₀ B complex vitamin–trace mineral tablet

Provides 418 kilocalories, 19.3 grams protein, 29.9 grams fat
See Table 4.4 in Chapter 4 for caloric needs of cats.

Provides phosphorus at 47 percent, potassium at 198 percent, sodium at 172 percent of a cat's daily needs. To feed this diet with a normal amount of phosphorus, substitute 3 bonemeal tablets for the 1¹/₂ calcium carbonate tablets.

Beef and Rice Diet (Low-protein, low-phosphorus, normal potassium, normal sodium diet providing 56.8 grams protein/1000 kilocalories)

4 ounces lean ground beef (raw weight), cooked

¹/₂ ounce clams, canned, chopped in juice

¹/₂ cup rice, long-grain, cooked

1 tablespoon chicken fat

1¹/₂ calcium carbonate tablets (600 milligrams calcium)

¹/₄ multiple vitamin-mineral tablet

¹/₁₀ B complex vitamin–trace mineral tablet

Provides 443 kilocalories, 25.2 grams protein, 26.6 grams fat
See Table 4.4 in Chapter 4 for caloric needs of cats.

Provides phosphorus at 52 percent, potassium at 123 percent, sodium at 206 percent of a cat's daily needs. To feed this diet with a normal amount of phosphorus, substitute 3 bonemeal tablets for the 1¹/₂ calcium carbonate tablets.

Beef and Rice Diet (Low-protein, low-phosphorus, normal potassium, normal sodium diet providing 44.3 grams protein/1000 kilocalories)

4 ounces lean ground beef (raw weight), cooked

½ ounce clams, canned, chopped in juice

½ cup rice, long-grain, cooked

2 tablespoons chicken fat

1½ calcium carbonate tablets (600 milligrams calcium)

¼ multiple vitamin-mineral tablet

¹/₁₀ B complex vitamin–trace mineral tablet

Provides 569 kilocalories, 25.2 grams protein, 40.5 grams fat
See Table 4.4 in Chapter 4 for caloric needs of cats.

Provides phosphorus at 45 percent, potassium at 105 percent, sodium at 175 percent of daily a cat's needs. To feed this diet with a normal amount of phosphorus, substitute 3 bonemeal tablets for the 1½ calcium carbonate tablets. Add ⅛ teaspoon potassium chloride to increase potassium content.

Beef Diet (Low-protein, low-phosphorus, normal potassium, normal sodium diet providing 55.3 grams protein/1000 kilocalories)

4 ounces lean ground beef (raw weight), cooked

½ ounce clams, canned, chopped in juice

5 teaspoons chicken fat

1 calcium carbonate tablet (400 milligrams calcium)

¹/₄ multiple vitamin-mineral tablet

¹/₁₀ B complex vitamin–trace mineral tablet

Provides 430 kilocalories, 23.8 grams protein, 35.8 grams fat
See Table 4.4 in Chapter 4 for caloric needs of cats.

Provides phosphorus at 50 percent, potassium at 126 percent, sodium at 234 percent of a cat's daily needs. To feed this diet with a normal amount of phosphorus, substitute 3 bonemeal tablets for the 1 calcium carbonate tablet. Add ¹/₈ teaspoon potassium chloride to increase potassium content.

Beef and Potato Diet (*Low-protein, low-phosphorus, normal potassium, normal sodium diet providing 46.7 grams protein/1000 kilocalories*)

4 ounces lean ground beef (raw weight), cooked

¹/₂ ounce clams, canned, chopped in juice

¹/₂ cup potato, boiled with skin

2 tablespoons chicken fat

1¹/₂ calcium carbonate tablets (400 milligrams calcium)

¹/₄ multiple vitamin-mineral tablet

¹/₁₀ B complex vitamin–trace mineral tablet

Provides 540 kilocalories, 25.2 grams protein, 40.5 grams fat
See Table 4.4 in Chapter 4 for caloric needs of cats.

Provides phosphorus at 46 percent, potassium at 194 percent, sodium at 185 percent of a cat's daily needs. To feed this diet with a normal amount of phosphorus, substitute 3 bonemeal tablets for the 1¹/₂ calcium carbonate tablets.

Tuna and Rice Diet (Low-protein, low-phosphorus, normal potassium, high-sodium diet providing 53.4 grams protein/1000 kilocalories)

3 ounces tuna, canned in water

½ ounce clams, canned, chopped in juice

½ cup rice, long-grain, cooked

2 tablespoons chicken fat

⅛ teaspoon salt substitute—potassium chloride

1½ calcium carbonate tablets (600 milligrams calcium)

¼ multiple vitamin-mineral tablet

⅒ B complex vitamin–trace mineral tablet

Provides 468 kilocalories, 25 grams protein, 30 grams fat
See Table 4.4 in Chapter 4 for caloric needs of cats.

Provides phosphorus at 50 percent and potassium at 190 percent of a cat's daily needs. Sodium depends on using low-salt tuna. To feed this diet with a normal amount of phosphorus, substitute 3 bonemeal tablets for the 1½ calcium carbonate tablets.

Tuna and Rice Diet (Low-protein, low-phosphorus, normal potassium, high-sodium diet providing 44.8 grams protein/1000 kilocalories)

2 ounces tuna, canned in water

½ ounce clams, canned, chopped in juice

⅓ cup rice, long-grain, cooked

2 tablespoons chicken fat

⅛ teaspoon salt substitute—potassium chloride

1 calcium carbonate tablet (400 milligrams calcium)

¼ multiple vitamin-mineral tablet

⅒ B complex vitamin–trace mineral tablet

Provides 406 kilocalories, 18.2 grams protein, 29.6 grams fat
See Table 4.4 in Chapter 4 for caloric needs of cats.

Provides phosphorus at 46 percent and potassium at 209 percent of cat's daily needs. Sodium depends on using low-salt tuna. To feed this diet with a normal amount of phosphorus, substitute 3 bonemeal tablets for the 1 calcium carbonate tablet.

Patient Evaluation during Dietary Management

The evaluation of all patients is done by periodic blood chemistry measurements and any other appropriate testing. It is expected that abnormal blood values will improve or return to normal. After recovery it becomes important to modify dietary restrictions to provide an animal's nutritional needs. Without this monitoring it is possible that nutrient deficiency could develop.

The owner-prepared diets offer more choices of special diet for disease conditions than are available from commercial pet food companies. An animal's specific needs can be met with owner-prepared diets. That might be possible if a commercial diet just happens to provide what is needed for recovery.

With improvement some of the fat-soluble vitamins can be given. It is not necessary to give them more than weekly or several times a month. The liver stores these vitamins, and it takes months or years to deplete the stores of vitamins A and D, vitamins that have the greatest potential for being toxic.

References

1. Brown, Scott A. 1994. Canine renal disease. In *The Waltham Book of Clinical Nutrition of the Dog and Cat*, edited by J.M. Wills and K.W. Simpson, 313–334. Oxford: Pergamon Press.

2. Moraillon, Robert and Roger Wolter. 1994. Feline renal disease. In *The Waltham Book of Clinical Nutrition of the Dog and Cat*, edited by J.M. Wills and K.W. Simpson, 277–291. Oxford: Pergamon Press.

3. Grauer, Gregory F. and India F. Lane. 1994. Acute renal failure: Strategies for its prevention. In *Nephrology and Urology*, Waltham Symposium Number 16, edited by C. Tony Buffington and James H. Sokolowski, 23–30. Vernon, Calif.: Kal Kan Foods.

4. Kopple, Joel D. 1991. Role of diet in the progression of chronic renal fail-

ure: Experience with human studies and proposed mechanisms by which nutrients may retard progression. *Journal Nutrition* 121(11S):S124.

5. Polzin, David J., Carl A. Osborne, and Larry G. Adams. 1991. Effect of modified protein diets in dogs and cats with chronic renal failure: Current status. *Journal of Nutrition* 121(11S):S140–S144.

6. Leibetseder, J. and K. Neufeld. 1991. *Effects of Dietary Protein and Phosphorus Levels in Dogs with Chronic Renal Failure.* Purina International Nutrition Symposium in Association with the Eastern States Veterinary Conference. 15 January, 35–38.

7. Polzin, David J. 1991. *Can Diet Modify Progression of Chronic Renal Failure?* Purina International Nutrition Symposium in Association with the Eastern States Veterinary Conference. 15 January, 29–33.

8. Lewis, Lon D., Mark L. Morris, and Michael S. Hand. 1987. *Small Animal Clinical Nutrition III,* 3d ed. Topeka: Mark Morris Associates, 1–15.

CHAPTER 14
Diet and Urinary Tract Stone Disease

Urinary calculi are common, with 1 to 3 percent of all dogs and cats suffering at some time. The most important cause in cats is dietary. Diet is a common cause in dogs, but urinary tract infection is a significant cause of some stones. Urinary calculi are more common in animals fed commercial pet foods.

Some urinary calculi grow so big that they remain in the bladder. Urinary calculi can also be small enough to pass into the urethra, and some can lodge there and obstruct urination. Urinary calculi cause signs of strangury, frequent urination, urinary incontinence, and hematuria. Urinary calculi can remain in the bladder for months before signs of a problem are recognized.

Cystic calculi can often be identified on abdominal palpation. Radiographs reveal most calculi; urate stones are radiolucent and are not revealed. Calculi the size of sand are not apparent on radiographs, but they can readily obstruct the urethra. Urinalysis can assist in evaluating for urinary tract calculi. Urinalysis cannot prove the presence of calculi, but it can reveal urinary tract infection and conditions conducive to calculi formation such as alkaline urine and crystal formation. Other tests are usually not necessary to evaluate for calculi.

Types of Urinary Tract Calculi[1,2]

In cats struvite calculi containing magnesium, phosphate, and ammonia or hydrogen are most common, representing 65 to 70 percent of all calculi. Calcium oxalate calculi are the second most common at 20 percent. The third most common calculi are urates, and calcium phosphate calculi compose the remainder.

Dogs are similar in that struvite calculi are most common. Calcium oxalate calculi are next in frequency, followed by cystine and urate calculi. Cystine calculi appear in some dogs with a genetic defect causing urinary excretion of excess cystine. Urate stones are common in dogs with a genetic difference (dalmatians) that causes purines to be metabolized to uric acid. In these dogs urinary excretion of uric acid often results in calculi formation.

Pathogenesis of Struvite Calculi[1,2]

■ Diet-Altered Acid-Base Balance and Disease

Acid-base alterations contribute significantly to the formation of urinary tract calculi. Some calculi result from urinary tract infection, but the diet is important for their formation in many dogs. Diet is the most important factor for calculi formation in cats. Until recently, the compositions of commercial cat foods favored the formation of calculi. Most cat foods have been modified to reduce the risk of calculi formation.

■ Urinary Tract Stones and Urolithiasis in Cats[2]

The incidence of urinary tract calculi formation in feline urologic syndrome has gradually increased during the past three decades. During that time cats have been confined more, and greater numbers have been fed commercial cat foods. When cats hunted for food or ate owner-prepared foods, feline urologic syndrome was uncommon.

Urinary tract infection plays no role in struvite calculi formation in cats, although it is the major cause in dogs. In the past, suggested causes in cats included infection, both bacterial and viral; early castration of males; endocrine imbalance; high dietary ash, magnesium, phosphate, and nitrogen; low water intake; obesity; dry cat foods; and stricter confinement of cats, causing less frequent urination.

Feline urologic syndrome is very uncommon in cats fed as carnivores. Dry commercial cat foods contain primarily vegetable material, however. Grain and soy products are the most abundant ingredients. These foods also contain mineral mixtures that often include calcium carbonate (promotes alkaline conditions) or bone (high in magnesium). Without special precautions a cat food based on these ingredients produces neutral or alkaline urine, a factor that contributes to feline urologic syndrome. The primary cause of feline urologic syndrome is now known to be the formation of neutral or alkaline urine in an animal that evolved to produce acidic urine. Carnivores consuming a high-protein meat diet produce acid urine, so cat foods require mineral compositions appropriate for producing acid urine.

In addition to protein, some dietary minerals such as calcium chloride and ammonium chloride promote acid formation. Dietary minerals containing sodium, potassium, magnesium, or even calcium produce alkaline conditions. Any chemical that readily decomposes to carbon dioxide and water generally causes body fluids to become more alkaline. After the carbon dioxide is excreted, the rest of the chemical remains and promotes the alkalinity.

■ Calculi Formation[3]

Many metabolic factors appear to be important in the formation of struvite calculi. Urinary concentrations of magnesium, ammonia, and phosphate are important, with calculi formation more likely with an increase in their concentrations. Any struvite formed remains in solution in acid urine. Struvite crystallizes to form insoluble calculi in alkaline or neutral urine. It has been believed that the magnesium content of diets is a factor in the formation of calculi. Under dietary conditions that produce a neutral urine pH, the major dietary factor that contributes to a high incidence of calculi is high magnesium. Under these same dietary conditions that produce a neutral urine pH, there are small effects on calculi formation from (1) variation in water intake and salt intake, (2) frequency of urination, and (3) dietary levels of calcium, phosphate, and other minerals. Some of these factors, plus others such as infection and level of ash, can affect urine pH. Decreasing the pH of urine not only prevents calculi formation but also dissolves calculi that have already formed.

In summary, struvite stone formation is associated with feeding diets that result in neutral to alkaline urine and is not primarily related to diets high in magnesium. Since the cat evolved as a desert animal, it efficiently conserves water and produces a concentrated urine. Concentrations are high for magnesium, ammonium, and phosphate that become supersaturated and form crystals at neutral and alkaline pH; the formation of struvite crystals and stones follows. At acid pH (below pH 6.6), struvite remains largely in solution, despite a high mineral content.

Feeding to Prevent Urinary Stones[3]

Diets for cats should have a composition that will produce an acid urine (pH should be 6.2 to 6.6) in cats fed free-choice. Diet directly affects urine pH for a number of hours after eating (Fig. 14.1).[4] A diet producing urine in the desired pH range should not result in a urine pH greater than 7.0 during any time four to six hours after feeding. However, the diet should not have the potential of reducing the pH too much because that can lead to demineralization of bones, resulting in osteoporosis. The urine pH of carnivores eating natural prey is between 6.2 and 6.6, so this pH should be safe, even for long-term feeding.

A diet that produces urine pH greater than 7.0 in an adult cat produces a much lower pH in a growing kitten. The urine pH during bone growth can be less than 6.0 until the animal is over a year old. That low

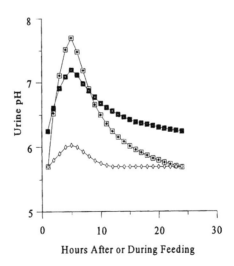

Figure 14.1. Changes in urine pH due to eating. Open squares = animals fed once a day. Shaded squares = animals fed ad libitum. Open diamonds = animals fed lower-pH diet once a day (adapted from Morris, 1995).

pH has no harmful effects during the cat's growth. If the diet continues to produce a low urine pH after growth stops, demineralization of bone will occur, leading to osteoporosis. The low urine pH in growing cats explains why struvite stone formation is rare until the animal is older than one year old; it is most common at three to four years of age.

Dietary Management of Struvite Calculi in Cats[3]

Cats with struvite calculi must be fed a diet that has little effect on increasing urine pH. Diets formulated with animal protein are most important in maintaining a low-urine pH.

Dietary magnesium has been thought to contribute to struvite calculi formation. That prompted manufacturers to reduce magnesium levels in cat foods. High dietary magnesium does not promote calculi formation, however. Magnesium is necessary for normal urinary calcium excretion. Reducing dietary magnesium can reduce calcium excretion and promote formation of calcium oxalate calculi. Humans with recurring oxalate stone formation have fewer recurrences when magnesium intake is increased. The following diets for cats have higher than usual magnesium concentrations. They do not contain the smaller amounts found in many commercial cat foods.

Since phosphate combines with magnesium to form struvite crystals, it is possible that controlling dietary phosphate might reduce calculi formation. However, feeding recommended phosphate levels to normal cats does not affect calculi formation. If anything, phosphate causes urine pH to become more acid, which reduces calculi formation. Commercial cat foods have acidifying agents added, such as phosphoric acid salts. This is comparable to medicating cats with acidifiers, which is not recommended. "No specific dosage of acidifier can be considered safe and effective under all conditions."[3] Consequently, natural sources of phosphate should be fed to acidify urine. Brewer's yeast is an important source of phosphate in the following cat diets.

Manufacturers produce low-ash cat foods so less ash must be excreted in urine. High-ash diets do not contribute to stone formation, however.

The following diets contain nutrients that maintain low urine pH and contain recommended levels of magnesium, phosphate, and ash for normal cats. For cats with struvite calculi, the recommended dietary level for magnesium is 20 to 40 milligrams/100 kilocalories and for phosphorus is 125 to 250 milligrams/100 kilocalories. These are both higher than National Research Council (NRC) recommendations for growing or adult cats. The levels of these two minerals increase with removal of dietary oil (where oil is included) and rice, something that reduces caloric content approximately 150 kilocalories. Dietary calcium levels follow NRC recommendations. Diets with higher sodium, formulated with sardines, tuna, or salmon, will increase water consumption. Increased water consumption helps prevent calculi formation.

Tofu and Sardines Diet

3¹/₃ ounces tofu, raw firm

2¹/₄ ounces sardines, canned, tomato sauce

¹/₂ yolk of egg, large, hard-boiled

¹/₂ ounce clams, canned, chopped in juice

¹/₃ cup brown rice, long-grain, cooked

2 teaspoons vegetable (canola) oil

¹/₂ ounce brewer's yeast

1 bonemeal tablet (10-grain or equivalent)

¹/₂ multiple vitamin-mineral tablet

Provides 501 kilocalories, 37.4 grams protein, 29.6 grams fat
See Table 4.4 in Chapter 4 for a cat's caloric needs. Provides 62.2 milligrams sodium/100-kilocalorie diet—a high-sodium intake

---

Tofu and Tuna Diet

3¹/₃ ounces tofu, raw firm

2 ounces tuna, canned in water, without added salt

¹/₂ yolk of egg, large, hard-boiled

½ ounce clams, canned, chopped in juice

⅓ cup brown rice, long-grain, cooked

½ ounce brewer's yeast

2 teaspoons vegetable (canola) oil

2 bonemeal tablets (10-grain or equivalent)

½ multiple vitamin-mineral tablet

Provides 446 kilocalories, 39.7 grams protein, 23 grams fat
See Table 4.4 in Chapter 4 for a cat's caloric needs. Provides
78.9 milligrams sodium/100-kilocalorie diet—a high-sodium
intake

Tofu and Salmon Diet

3⅓ ounces tofu, raw firm

2 ounces salmon, canned with bone

½ yolk of egg, large, hard-boiled

½ ounce clams, canned, chopped in juice

⅓ cup brown rice, long-grain, cooked

½ ounce brewer's yeast

2 teaspoons vegetable (canola) oil

1 bonemeal tablet (10-grain or equivalent)

½ multiple vitamin-mineral tablet

Provides 482 kilocalories, 39.7 grams protein, 26.5 grams fat
See Table 4.4 in Chapter 4 for a cat's caloric needs. Provides
79.2 milligrams sodium/100-kilocalorie diet—a high-sodium
intake

Tofu and Chicken Diet

3¹/₃ ounces tofu, raw firm

2²/₃ ounces chicken breast (raw weight), cooked

¹/₂ yolk of egg, large, hard-boiled

¹/₂ ounce clams, canned, chopped in juice

¹/₃ cup brown rice, long-grain, cooked

¹/₂ ounce brewer's yeast

2 teaspoons vegetable (canola) oil

2 bonemeal tablets (10-grain or equivalent)

¹/₂ multiple vitamin-mineral tablet

Provides 469 kilocalories, 42.6 grams protein, 23.6 grams fat
See Table 4.4 in Chapter 4 for a cat's caloric needs. Provides 18.3 milligrams sodium/100-kilocalorie diet—a low sodium intake

---

Tofu and Beef Diet

3¹/₃ ounces tofu, raw firm

4 ounces lean ground beef (raw weight), cooked

¹/₂ yolk of egg, large, hard-boiled

¹/₂ ounce clams, canned, chopped in juice

¹/₃ cup brown rice, long-grain, cooked

¹/₂ ounce brewer's yeast

2 bonemeal tablets (10-grain or equivalent)

¹/₂ multiple vitamin-mineral tablet

Provides 494 kilocalories, 46.7 grams protein, 24.1 grams fat
See Table 4.4 in Chapter 4 for a cat's caloric needs. Provides 20.2 milligrams sodium/100-kilocalorie diet—a low sodium intake

Tofu and Lamb Diet

$3^1/_3$ *ounces tofu, raw firm*

4 ounces lean ground lamb (raw weight), cooked

$^1/_2$ *yolk of egg, large, hard-boiled*

$^1/_2$ *ounce clams, canned, chopped in juice*

$^1/_3$ *cup brown rice, long-grain, cooked*

$^1/_2$ *ounce brewer's yeast*

2 bonemeal tablets (10-grain or equivalent)

$^1/_2$ *multiple vitamin-mineral tablet*

Provides 522 kilocalories, 46.5 grams protein, 27.4 grams fat
See Table 4.4 in Chapter 4 for a cat's caloric needs. Provides
16.2 milligrams sodium/100-kilocalorie diet—a low sodium
intake

Tofu and Clams Diet

$^3/_4$ *cup tofu, raw firm*

$^1/_2$ *yolk of egg, large, hard-boiled*

1 ounce clams, canned, chopped in juice

$^1/_3$ *cup brown rice, long-grain, cooked*

$^1/_2$ *ounce brewer's yeast*

1 tablespoon vegetable (canola) oil

1 bonemeal tablet (10-grain or equivalent)

$^1/_2$ *multiple vitamin-mineral tablet*

Provides 548 kilocalories, 45.8 grams protein, 34.6 grams fat
See Table 4.4 in Chapter 4 for a cat's caloric needs. Provides
13.8 milligrams sodium/100-kilocalorie diet—a low sodium
intake

If rice is eliminated from any of these diets, the caloric content will be 68 calories less, and the protein content will be about 1 gram less. Without rice in beef or lamb diets, bonemeal is reduced to 1 tablet.

Dietary Management of Struvite Calculi in Dogs[3]

Dogs develop struvite calculi when their urine is alkaline and is saturated with magnesium and phosphate. Dogs must also have a urinary tract infection for struvite calculi formation. Sometimes bacteria cannot be cultured from urine or struvite calculi. Infection is still necessary for most struvite calculi formations. The infection responsible for calculi formation may have been eliminated by antibiotics. Also, infection can be present where it is not possible to culture and find bacteria. Some dogs produce alkaline urine despite being fed diets or drugs to acidify urine. These dogs also can develop struvite calculi without infection.

Diets containing reduced amounts of high-quality proteins, phosphorus, and magnesium reduce urea, phosphate, and magnesium in urine. Studies show these diets promote struvite stones' dissolution in dogs. All dogs in these studies also received antibiotics for urinary tract infection, however. Pet food manufacturers producing diets with low protein, magnesium, and phosphorus claim the diets are responsible for calculi dissolution. However, antibiotic treatment is far more responsible. If antibiotics are not given, calculi remain. If a dog with calculi receives antibiotics and no special diet, the calculi dissolve and disappear. Thus, diet is not critical for managing struvite calculi in dogs.

The following diets contain proper amounts of nutrients for meeting dogs' needs. The diets contain near normal levels of nutrients such as magnesium because reduction of this mineral can increase risk for calcium oxalate stones. Sodium chloride can be increased to promote a greater intake of water.

Cottage Cheese and Rice Diet

⅔ cup cottage cheese, 2 percent fat

1 egg, large, hard-boiled

2 cups brown rice, long-grain, cooked

2 teaspoons vegetable (canola) oil

½ ounce brewer's yeast

4 bonemeal tablets (10-grain or equivalent)

¼ teaspoon salt substitute—potassium chloride

1 multiple vitamin-mineral tablet

Provides 780 kilocalories, 42.9 grams protein, 22 grams fat
Supports caloric needs of a 25- to 26-pound dog
Provides 92 milligrams sodium/100-kilocalorie diet—a high sodium intake

Beef and Rice Diet

¼ pound very lean beef (raw weight), cooked

1 egg, large, hard-boiled

2 cups brown rice, long-grain, cooked

½ ounce brewer's yeast

4 bonemeal tablets (10-grain or equivalent)

¼ teaspoon salt substitute—potassium chloride

1 multiple vitamin-mineral tablet

Provides 730 kilocalories, 40.7 grams protein, 19.7 grams fat
Supports caloric needs of a 24-pound dog
Provides 21.8 milligrams sodium/100-kilocalorie diet—a low sodium intake

---

Tuna and Rice Diet

4 ounces tuna, canned in water, without added salt

1 egg, large, hard-boiled

2 cups brown rice, long-grain, cooked

2 teaspoons vegetable (canola) oil

½ ounce brewer's yeast

4 bonemeal tablets (10-grain or equivalent)

¼ teaspoon salt substitute—potassium chloride

1 multiple vitamin-mineral tablet

Provides 760 kilocalories, 47.3 grams protein, 21.1 grams fat
Supports caloric needs of a 31-pound dog
Provides 92.7 milligrams sodium/100-kilocalorie diet—a high sodium intake. Without the 2 teaspoons vegetable oil, the caloric content is 670 kilocalories, and fat content is 24 grams. The oil can be omitted from the diet if the plan is to reduce fat intake.

Dietary Management of Calcium Oxalate Calculi in Cats and Dogs[5,6]

Calcium oxalate calculi develop because urine is saturated with calcium and oxalate. Found in many foods, oxalate is a carbohydrate that can be produced from carbohydrate-like chemicals in foods. Inhibitors of oxalate calculi formation include phosphorus, magnesium, and citrate. Oxalate stones form more readily in acid urine, but urine with low pH and high calcium concentrations does not produce calcium oxalate calculi when urine magnesium is normal or increased. Thus, dietary magnesium is important for preventing calcium oxalate calculi formation.

Most pets are fed commercial pet foods prior to forming calcium oxalate calculi. After surgical removal of these calculi, about 50 percent of pets once more form calculi within three years. Therefore, a different kind of diet must be fed to prevent any recurrence.

The following diets contain low oxalate and minimum calcium.

They also contain normal phosphorus, which prevents absorption of excess calcium. The diet should contain no more than minimum vitamin D to minimize absorption of dietary calcium. Diets for cats must promote acid urine, but that may be less important for dogs. Most importantly the following diets provide enough magnesium to minimize calculi formation. Magnesium should be 20 to 40 milligrams/100 kilocalories of diet. High dietary sodium increases urine calcium, prompting some to recommend reducing dietary salt. It is unknown whether this promotes calculi formation, however. Anything increasing water consumption reduces stone recurrence. Current recommendations are to feed a vegetarian-type high-fiber diet that is low in oxalate, calcium, and vitamin D. The pet should also not be given excess amounts of substances, such as vitamin C, that can be converted to oxalate.

■ **Adult Dogs with Oxalate Stones**

Black-Eyed Peas and Rice Diet

⅔ cup black-eyed peas, boiled

2 cups brown rice, long-grain, cooked

1 tablespoon vegetable (canola) oil

2 bonemeal tablets (10-grain or equivalent)

¼ teaspoon salt substitute—potassium chloride

1 multiple vitamin-mineral tablet

¹/₁₀ teaspoon table salt (sodium chloride)

Provides 696 kilocalories, 19.3 grams protein, 17.8 grams fat
Supports caloric needs of a 21- to 22-pound dog
Provides calcium at 55 percent, phosphorus at 102 percent, sodium at 33 percent, vitamin D at 63 percent of requirements

Black-Eyed Peas and Potato Diet

1 cup black-eyed peas, boiled

2 cups potato, cooked with skin

1 tablespoon vegetable (canola) oil

2 bonemeal tablets (10-grain or equivalent)

1 multiple vitamin-mineral tablet

¹/₁₀ teaspoon table salt (sodium chloride)

Provides 598 kilocalories, 19.4 grams protein, 14.6 grams fat
Supports caloric needs of a 17- to 18-pound dog
Provides calcium at 61 percent, phosphorus at 98 percent, sodium at 34 percent, vitamin D at 70 percent of requirements

■ Adult Cats with Oxalate Stones

Tuna Diet

4 ounces tuna, canned in water, without added salt

¹/₂ yolk of egg, large, hard-boiled

1 tablespoon vegetable (canola) oil

¹/₄ bonemeal tablet (10-grain or equivalent)

Provides 273 kilocalories, 26.61 grams protein, 18.6 grams fat
See Table 4.4 in Chapter 4 for a cat's caloric needs.
Provides calcium at 31 percent, phosphorus at 97 percent, vitamin D at 193 percent of requirements. Sodium is high and depends on sodium content of tuna.

Tuna and Rice Diet

4 ounces tuna, canned in water, without added salt

½ yolk of egg, large, hard-boiled

⅓ cup rice, long-grain, cooked

1 tablespoon vegetable (canola) oil

1 bonemeal tablet (10-grain or equivalent)

Provides 342 kilocalories, 28 grams protein, 18.8 grams fat
See Table 4.4 in Chapter 4 for a cat's caloric needs.
Provides calcium at 60 percent and phosphorus at 98 percent of requirements. Sodium is high and depends on sodium content of tuna. Vitamin D is low.

Salmon and Rice Diet

4⅓ ounces salmon, canned with bone, low-salt

½ yolk of egg, large, hard-boiled

½ ounce clams, canned, chopped in juice

⅓ cup rice, long-grain, cooked

2 teaspoons vegetable (canola) oil

Provides 399 kilocalories, 31.7 grams protein, 22.2 grams fat
See Table 4.4 in Chapter 4 for a cat's caloric needs.
Provides calcium at 66 percent and phosphorus at 140 percent of requirements. Sodium is high and depends on sodium content of tuna. Vitamin D is low.

Dietary Management of Urate Calculi in Cats and Dogs[7]

Urate and uric acid calculi form because ammonium urate and uric acid crystallize in urine. Urates and uric acid are produced by degradation of purine nucleotides involved in cell division and protein manufacture. Normally the liver degrades these substances to compounds that the kidneys readily excrete. In dalmatians, the liver converts only 30 to 40 percent of urates to the excretable form. This leaves considerable uric acid to be excreted. Many dalmatians show no clinical problems, but some form urinary crystals and calculi from high uric acid levels in urine. Some other breeds do not degrade urates to the readily excretable form because liver disease compromises this function. Some of these animals form urate calculi.

A predictable number of dalmatians develop urate calculi, and many are treated with drugs. Allopurinol is routinely used to reduce formation of urates from purines. This drug must be given daily, and it can have side effects. Forty years ago when drugs were not available to prevent urate calculi, low-purine diets were fed. Faithful feeding of these diets prevented calculi formation. On feeding purine-containing foods, urate stones recurred, however. The following diets are low in purines and are preferable to drugs for managing urate calculi disease.

Dogs with liver disease and urate calculi may require diets with lower protein in addition to low purines. These dogs often have elevated blood and urine ammonia because the liver cannot efficiently convert ammonia to urea. Although it may be necessary to feed a low-protein diet, dogs with liver disease often have a need for normal amounts of protein. Reducing dietary protein can cause complications from a protein deficiency. For example, low dietary protein can cause hypoproteinemia.

These diets are more effective in preventing calculi recurrence if they promote greater water consumption. Urate crystals do not form in dilute urine as readily as they do in concentrated urine. Urate calculi are also more soluble in alkaline than in acid urine. The following diets produce an alkaline ash and urine.

It is necessary to add taurine to the diets for cats with urate stones. Foods rich in taurine also contain high amounts of purines; they cannot be used.

■ Adult Dogs with Urate Calculi

Cottage Cheese and Potato Diet

²/₃ *cup cottage cheese, 2 percent fat*

2 cups potato, cooked with skin

1 tablespoon vegetable (canola) oil

½ calcium carbonate tablet (200 milligrams calcium)

2 bonemeal tablets (10-grain or equivalent)

1 multiple vitamin-mineral tablet

Provides 531 kilocalories, 26.5 grams protein, 17.3 grams fat
Supports caloric needs of a 14- to 15-pound dog

Cottage Cheese and Rice Diet

²/₃ *cup cottage cheese, 2 percent fat*

2 cups rice, long-grain, cooked

1 tablespoon vegetable (canola) oil

½ calcium carbonate tablet (200 milligrams calcium)

3 bonemeal tablets (10-grain or equivalent)

¼ teaspoon salt substitute—potassium chloride

1 multiple vitamin-mineral tablet

Provides 672 kilocalories, 29.2 grams protein, 18 grams fat
Supports caloric needs of a 20- to 21-pound dog

■ Adult Cats with Urate Calculi

Cottage Cheese and Potato Diet

²/₃ *cup cottage cheese, 2 percent fat*

1 cup potato, cooked with skin

1 tablespoon vegetable (canola) oil

2 bonemeal tablets (10-grain or equivalent)

¹/₂ *multiple vitamin-mineral tablet*

50 milligrams taurine

Provides 397 kilocalories, 23.7 grams protein, 17.3 grams fat
See Table 4.4 in Chapter 4 for a cat's caloric needs.

Cottage Cheese and Rice Diet

²/₃ *cup cottage cheese, 2 percent fat*

³/₄ *cup rice, long-grain, cooked*

1 tablespoon vegetable (canola) oil

2 bonemeal tablets (10-grain or equivalent)

¹/₄ *teaspoon salt substitute—potassium chloride*

¹/₂ *multiple vitamin-mineral tablet*

50 milligrams taurine

Provides 413 kilocalories, 23.9 grams protein, 17.4 grams fat
See Table 4.4 in Chapter 4 for a cat's caloric needs.

Dietary Management of Cystine Calculi in Dogs[1]

Cystine stones form because of a genetic defect that causes excess urinary excretion of cystine. Signs of cystine calculi do not appear before the dog is three to five years old. Treatment is surgical removal; however, the recurrence rate is high, which makes prevention important. There is no proven successful means for preventing calculi reformation. Protein-restricted and low-methionine diets and increasing urine production might help. The following diet restricts protein and promotes urine production.

Tofu and Potato Diet

1½ ounces tofu, raw firm

2 cups potato, cooked with skin

2 tablespoons vegetable (canola) oil

¼ teaspoon salt substitute—potassium chloride

4 bonemeal tablets (10-grain or equivalent)

1 multiple vitamin-mineral tablet

Provides 584 kilocalories, 12.7 grams protein (meets 100 percent of recommended requirement), 32.2 grams fat

Supports caloric needs of a 17- to 18-pound dog

Provides 101 percent of protein and 166 percent of methionine requirements

Add ⅛ teaspoon table salt to increase water intake.

Feline Idiopathic Lower–Urinary Tract Disease[8]

Straining to urinate and voiding small amounts frequently, often with blood, are signs of urinary tract obstruction in cats. A great number of both males and females are not obstructed with calculi, however. Most cats with these signs and no obstruction have idiopathic lower–urinary tract disease for which a complete workup shows no cause. Almost 1 percent of all cats in the United States show signs of urinary tract obstruction, and of those the majority suffer not from stone formation but from the idiopathic nonobstructive problem, making it the most common cause of clinical signs of lower–urinary tract disease. The incidence of this problem in clinical female cats is 58 percent and in males 79 percent.

Cats with idiopathic lower urinary tract disease are far more likely to be fed dry commercial cat food than are nonaffected cats. Affected cats do not respond to medical management. Their diet must be changed. Feeding a canned commercial cat food solves the problem. Feeding any one of the diets in this book to cats affected with lower–urinary tract disease also solves the problem.

References

1. Hoppe, Astrid E. 1994. Canine lower urinary tract disease. In *The Waltham Book of Clinical Nutrition of the Dog and Cat*, edited by J.M. Wills and K.W. Simpson, 335–352. Oxford: Pergamon Press.

2. Markwell, Peter J. and C. Tony Buffington. 1994. Feline lower urinary tract disease. In *The Waltham Book of Clinical Nutrition of the Dog and Cat*, edited by J.M. Wills and K.W. Simpson, 293–311. Oxford: Pergamon Press.

3. Buffington, C. Tony. 1992. Nutritional aspects of struvite urolithiasis in dogs and cats. In *Nephrology and Urology*, Waltham Symposium Number 16, edited by C. Tony Buffington and James H. Sokolowski, 51–57. Vernon, Calif.: Kal Kan Foods.

4. Morris, James G. 1995. *Nutrition and Nutritional Diseases in Animals*. 18-1 to 18-11. Class Notes for Veterinary Medicine 408, School of Veterinary Medicine, University of California, Davis.

5. Lulich, Jody P., Carl A. Osborne, Larry J. Felice, David J. Polzin, Rosama Thumchai, and Sherry Sanderson. 1992. Calcium oxalate urolithiasis. In *Nephrology and Urology*, Waltham Symposium Number 16, edited by C. Tony Buffington and James H. Sokolowski, 69–74. Vernon, Calif.: Kal Kan Foods.

6. Kirk, Claudia A., Gerald V. Ling, Charles E. Franti, and Janet M. Scarlett. 1995. Evaluation of factors associated with development of calcium oxalate urolithiasis in cats. *Journal of the American Veterinary Medical Association* 207:1429–1434.

7. Senior, David F. 1992. Urate urolithiasis. In *Nephrology and Urology*, Waltham Symposium Number 16, edited by C. Tony Buffington and James H. Sokolowski, 59–67. Vernon, Calif.: Kal Kan Foods.

8. Buffington, C. Tony, Dennis J. Chew, Michael S. Kendall, Peter V. Scrivani, Steven B. Thompson, Jean L. Blaisdell, and Bruce E. Woodworth. 1997. Clinical evaluation of cats with nonobstructive urinary tract diseases. *Journal of the American Veterinary Medical Association* 210:46–50.

CHAPTER 15
Diet and Endocrine Disease

Dogs and cats develop many endocrine diseases. Dietary management is unimportant for some diseases but for others is very important.

Thyroid Gland Diseases[1,2]

Hyperthyroidism has become a common disease of older cats. There is evidence that feline hyperthyroidism results from feeding commercial pet foods. Caused by a tumor or nodule of hyperactive tissue in the thyroid gland, it is a new disease in cats (appearing after 1970). Hyperthyroidism appeared with the feeding of canned cat foods. The disease has not occurred in developed countries where owners have not fed canned cat food, but with the switch to feeding canned cat food, the problem is appearing there. It is unknown how canned cat foods cause this thyroid abnormality.

If hyperthyroidism was an insignificant disease, the feeding of cat canned pet foods could continue. The disease is serious, however. Besides losing weight and having a continuous problem with diarrhea, affected cats manifest personality changes so that many do not remain enjoyable pets. Cost of treatment is usually high and is not always successful; some cases are fatal. Treatment of the problem can be life threatening. Medical management must include diets to restore weight. Feeding an owner-prepared diet is recommended to prevent hyperthyroidism.

Hypothyroidism usually results in weight gain. Hypothyroidism results from thyroid gland atrophy or inflammation. Management is based on administering thyroxine. Dietary management often includes reducing food intake to correct obesity.

Adrenal Gland Diseases[1,2]

Hyperadrenocorticism, or Cushing's disease, results in excess cortisol production. Treatment is to medically or surgically reduce cortisol release. Affected animals are also at risk for developing diabetes in part because they develop resistance to insulin. Dietary management can be important when it is also necessary to treat diabetes mellitus.

Adrenal gland destruction results in cortisol deficiency, or Addison's disease. Treatment is to replace cortisol. Dietary management is not necessary. Salt intake can be increased but is not necessary when proper amounts of hormone are given.

Parathyroid Gland Diseases[1,2]

Hyperparathyroidism releasing increased parathormone can be primary or secondary. Primary is usually caused by a parathyroid tumor. One secondary cause is feeding diets containing low calcium and normal phosphorus. Feeding all-meat diets without a calcium supplement causes this secondary, or nutritional, hyperparathyroidism. Thirty to 40 years ago commercial all-meat pet foods were not supplemented with calcium, and the problem was common. Since then all commercial diets have enough calcium to prevent hyperparathyroidism. The diets in this book contain National Research Council (NRC) recommended amounts of calcium. There are some exceptions, however. Diets to prevent calcium oxalate calculi contain lower calcium.

Parathyroid hormone deficiency is uncommon. Causes include parathyroid gland destruction or atrophy and surgery to remove parathyroid tumors that leaves little or no normal tissue. The spontaneous causes can be treated with vitamin D and calcium. Normal blood calcium shows treatment was successful.

Diabetes Mellitus[1,2]

Diabetes mellitus causes hyperglycemia by insulin deficiency and glucagon excess. Insulin is produced only in pancreatic islet cells. Glucagon is produced by pancreatic and small intestinal hormone–producing cells. Increased blood glucose or amino acids stimulate insulin release, which inhibits lipolysis in adipose tissue and protein catabolism in muscle. Insulin also inhibits conversion of fat and protein to glucose. Insulin promotes storage of fat, protein, and carbohydrate. Inadequate insulin results in hyperglycemia because gluconeogenesis is uninhibited and cells need insulin to take up glucose. An energy deficiency exists, causing fat to be mobilized from adipose stores. Circulating fat is removed by the liver and converted to ketone bodies for use as an alternate source of energy. The large amount of fat released cannot be metabolized completely, and the liver must store some. Eventually fat accumulations result in hepatic lipidosis.

Diabetes mellitus is managed by insulin and diets to correct metabolic abnormalities. Islet cells normally release insulin at rates responding to subtle blood glucose changes. Insulin given by injection once or twice daily cannot compare with the changing minute to minute release from a normal pancreas. Thus, diabetic patients are never well regulated, even though they may respond to treatment favorably and appear normal. The well-managed diabetic patient will have hepatic lipidosis despite treatment.

Diabetics can be regulated dietarily, but diets cannot replace insulin, which is almost always required. Insulin needs depend on diabetes type. With insulin-dependent diabetes mellitus, little or no insulin is produced because islets cells have been destroyed by autoimmune antibodies, drugs, toxins, or inflammation. Another group of diabetics produces insulin but not enough to meet normal or increased needs. In some cases insulin may be antagonized by female reproductive hormones or excess cortisone.

■ Diagnosis of Diabetes Mellitus[1,2]

Persistent hyperglycemia identifies diabetes mellitus. Glycosuria suggests diabetes mellitus. Glycosuria is also found in animals with no diabetes mellitus. Sometimes diabetes mellitus must be proven by measuring blood insulin or glucose after the patient is given glucose.

■ Dietary Management of Diabetes Mellitus[1-3]

Insulin Therapy
Dietary management of diabetes mellitus is important for animals with complete and partial insulin dependency. With complete dependency the proper diet must be fed when blood insulin peaks. With par-

tial dependency insulin requirements can be lowered with proper dietary management.

Insulin is available in short-acting and intermediate-acting forms. Regular insulin is short-acting and used primarily for hospitalized patients. Intermediate-acting forms are NPH (isophane insulin suspension), Lente, and mixtures of NPH and regular insulins.

Time of feeding after insulin injection is critical. A decision must also be made about feeding once a day or more often. Anorectic or unfed diabetic animals should receive some insulin to reduce fat catabolism. Blood testing during insulin therapy and feeding gives information on how to best manage the frequency of insulin administrations and feeding.

Diet Composition

Older wisdom held that a diabetic's diet should be low in carbohydrates. This is no longer considered correct. Diabetic dogs should be fed a diet high in complex carbohydrates (starch and dietary fiber that provide 50 to 55 percent of total energy), containing no simple sugars such as sucrose, restricted in fat (providing less than 20 percent of energy), and moderate in protein (providing 14 to 30 percent of energy).

As mentioned above it is almost impossible to regulate diabetics because optimal amounts of insulin are not always available. Dietary complex carbohydrates can improve this regulation.

Cats are not designed to eat a diet containing 50 percent complex carbohydrates. There is also no evidence that any special diet is of benefit in managing a cat with diabetes mellitus. Thus, this chapter has no recipes for feeding cats with diabetes.

Carbohydrates—The Source of Energy

Carbohydrate is the preferred source for energy in dogs. Digestion and absorption of selected carbohydrates can be slow. This prevents absorption of large amounts, which worsens hyperglycemia, and it causes fewer wide fluctuations in blood glucose. Also, a diet high in carbohydrates appears to increase the sensitivity of cells to insulin and improves their glucose uptake, thereby relieving hyperglycemia.

Complex Carbohydrates

The digestion of one complex carbohydrate, starch, is usually never complete. Rice starch is an exception. Feeding more poorly digested starches results in slower digestion and absorption so that blood glucose fluctuates less than with feeding readily digested carbohydrates. Sugar results in blood glucose fluctuating the most.

Fiber is another form of complex carbohydrate, but it is not digested and enters the colon. Dietary fiber helps control diabetes by promoting weight loss, slowing carbohydrate digestion, slowing glucose absorption, and reducing blood glucose fluctuations following a meal.

Dietary fiber has properties of being soluble or insoluble and fermentable or nonfermentable. Soluble fibers take up water and form gels. They slow gastric emptying, reduce nutrient absorption, and increase intestinal transit. Insoluble fibers take up little or no water and have a smaller effect on reducing digestion and absorption of a meal. Fibers that can be fermented are broken down by colonic bacteria. Fermentable fiber provides nutrients: short chain fatty acids.

Both soluble and insoluble fiber benefit diabetic dogs. Guar gum, one form of soluble fiber, sprinkled on food at levels of 8 grams/400 kilocalories reduces hyperglycemia in both normal and diabetic dogs for at least four hours after feeding. An insoluble fiber, wheat bran, has a similar but less pronounced effect at levels of 8 grams/400 kilocalories of diet. Feeding greater amounts of soluble fiber such as guar or pectin causes diarrhea in dogs. Feeding larger amounts of insoluble fiber such as wheat bran has little effect on dogs other than possibly reducing a diet's palatability.

Current recommendations are to feed a combination of soluble and insoluble fiber. Of the two the soluble is more important and more effective; less soluble than insoluble fiber is needed to achieve the same desired effect. The combination can reduce blood glucose fluctuations in diabetics eating regular diets and receiving daily injections of insulin.

There is no evidence that additional fiber is of any benefit in managing a cat with diabetes mellitus. Cats also do not readily accept a high-fiber diet.

■ Diets for Dogs with Diabetes Mellitus

High-Fiber, High-Carbohydrate, and Low-Fat Diet

1¹/₄ cups oatmeal or rolled oats, cooked

3¹/₂ ounces (¹/₄ cup) kidney beans, canned

1 egg, large, hard-boiled

1 cup mixed vegetables, cooked and drained

1¹/₂ calcium carbonate tablets (600 milligrams calcium)

1 multiple vitamin-mineral tablet

Provides 452 kilocalories, 24.5 grams protein, 8.9 grams fat
Supports caloric needs of a 12- to 13-pound dog

High-Fiber, High-Carbohydrate, and Low-Fat Diet

¹/₃ pound poultry breast (raw weight), cooked

2 cups potato, cooked with skin

Egg yolk of 1 egg, large, hard-boiled

¹/₂ cup mixed vegetables, cooked and drained

30 grams (1 ounce) wheat bran

2 calcium carbonate tablets (800 milligrams calcium)

1 multiple vitamin-mineral tablet

Provides 512 kilocalories, 45.8 grams protein, 10.2 grams fat
Supports caloric needs of a 14- to 15-pound dog

References

1. Maskell, Ian E. and Peter A. Graham. 1994. Endocrine disorders. In *The Waltham Book of Clinical Nutrition of the Dog and Cat*, edited by J.M. Wills and K.W. Simpson, 373–393. Oxford: Pergamon Press.

2. Peterson, Mark E. and Thomas K. Graves. Diagnosis and treatment of occult hyperthyroidism in cats. In *Endocrinology*, 15th Waltham Symposium, edited by Dennis J. Chew and James H. Sokolowske, 7–12. Vernon, Calif.: Kal Kan Foods.

3. Bauer, John E. and Ian E. Maskell. 1994. Dietary fibre: Perspectives in clinical management. In *The Waltham Book of Clinical Nutrition of the Dog and Cat*, edited by J.M. Wills and K.W. Simpson, 87–104. Oxford: Pergamon Press.

CHAPTER 16
Diet and Heart Disease

Heart disease is common in dogs and cats, especially in older animals. As many as 10 percent of all dogs have heart disease. Until the 1980s little was known about any relationship between diet and heart disease. Since then some important nutrients have been documented as important in preventing several forms of heart disease. Also, as has been known for years, nutrition is important in managing fluid retention caused by chronic heart failure.

Taurine and Heart Disease[1]

The amino acid taurine is essential for normal structure and function of the retina, platelets, and heart. With taurine deficiency, cats can develop feline taurine-deficient dilated cardiomyopathy. The problem can be suspected from a physical examination and thoracic radiographs showing heart enlargement. The problem is diagnosed by low plasma taurine (less that 20 micromoles/liter). Normal plasma taurine ranges between 50 and 120 micromoles/liter. Dilated cardiomyopathy also affects some American cocker spaniels, which have low plasma levels of both taurine and L-carnitine (see below). Heart disease in other animals may be related to a deficiency of these nutrients.

Most animals make enough taurine that deficiencies don't develop. Cats cannot make enough to meet their needs, however. Cats depend on dietary taurine to supply adequate amounts. Diets containing animal proteins usually provide cats with enough taurine. There are some exceptions. Animal proteins in cheese and eggs contain little or no taurine. Cats cannot be fed these proteins unless they are supplemented with taurine. Plants also do not manufacture taurine, so plant proteins in tofu or other soy products, beans, and cereals cannot be fed without taurine supplements. Plant-produced proteins can be fed to dogs because they produce taurine from other amino acids.

Taurine, unlike other amino acids, is not incorporated in protein structure but is free in body fluids. Meat processing that results in loss of its juices causes loss of taurine. Feeding processed nutrients can cause taurine deficiencies in cats.

Feline taurine-deficient dilated cardiomyopathy was not recognized before cats were fed commercial pet foods. Cats living primarily on a carnivorous diet do not develop the problem; they consume enough taurine. Since the pet food industry recognized that taurine deficiency was a cause of medical problems, it has supplemented cat foods with taurine. The first problem recognized was blindness caused by retinal degeneration. Addition of taurine to the diet solved that problem. Not enough taurine was added to prevent cardiomyopathies, however. With the recognition that heart problems were caused by taurine deficiency, more taurine was added to cat diets. Dry foods need high taurine, 1000 to 1200 milligrams taurine/kilogram dry weight. Canned foods need twice this amount to maintain normal taurine in body tissues.

Cats with cardiomyopathy are treated with taurine and given initial doses of 250 to 500 milligrams twice a day. If heart disease resolves, 6 to 12 weeks of therapy are required. (Other medications such as diuretics and vasodilators are also needed.) With improvement, taurine supplementation can be reduced to 250 milligrams daily. Recovered cats' diets should always contain adequate taurine.

Despite awareness of problems caused by taurine deficiency, some owners may feed cats inadequate taurine, especially if the cats' diets contain primarily cereals or a single processed food. It is unknown if all commercial cat foods contain adequate taurine. All diets for feeding normal cats in Chapter 5 contain enough taurine. Vegetarian diets have taurine added in a powder or capsule form.

Carnitine and Heart Disease[1]

Animals use lysine and methionine to synthesize L-carnitine. This compound is classified as a water-soluble vitamin or a nonessential amino acid. It is needed to transport free fatty acids into the mitochondria of cardiac muscle. Carnitine is esterified with fatty acids to facilitate their movement across cell membranes. Inside mitochondria, oxidation of fatty acids generates energy in the form of ATP. Carnitine remaining after fat oxidation forms esters with potentially toxic waste products and transports them from the mitochondria.

Carnitine deficiency is associated with heart problems in some boxer, Doberman pinscher, and American cocker spaniel dogs with dilated cardiomyopathy. Some of these dogs improve and live longer with oral L-carnitine supplements.

No one knows why some animals suffer from carnitine deficiency. It may result from inadequate dietary carnitine, lysine, or methionine or from intestinal malabsorption of these nutrients. Deficiency could also result from excess renal loss of these nutrients. Defective transport of carnitine esters across mitochondrial membranes could be a factor.

Carnitine deficiency is often difficult to diagnose. Dilated cardiomyopathy causes specific physical findings and radiographic changes. They do not prove carnitine deficiency, however. Plasma carnitine can be measured, but that can be normal and not necessarily reflect carnitine levels in cardiac muscle. Up to 80 percent of dogs with carnitine deficiency in cardiac muscle have normal or increased plasma carnitine concentrations. Deficiency is proven only by measuring carnitine in cardiac muscle biopsies.

Carnitine deficiency is treated with L-carnitine given orally at a dose of two grams mixed with food three times a day. This treatment appears to have few adverse side effects. With success, appetite and activity improve after one to four weeks of therapy. Carnitine supplementation increases its level in heart muscle in most, but not all, dogs.

Dilated cardiomyopathy caused by carnitine deficiency may be prevented by feeding diets high in carnitine. Carnitine is most abundant in red meat and dairy products. Feeding nonmeat-based commercial pet food results in dogs having plasma carnitine levels 50 percent lower than in those consuming meat-based diets. Thus, although dogs are said not to be strictly carnivores and they can be fed vegetarian diets, feeding the cereal-based commercial dog foods is not likely to support adequate carnitine levels in heart muscle. Furthermore, heat may inactivate carnitine, something possible during processing of commercial dog food.

Dilated cardiac myopathy caused by carnitine deficiency is prevented and treated best by feeding foods high in L-carnitine. The meat- and dairy product–based diets in Chapter 5 provide dogs with abundant carnitine.

Hypertension, Sodium, Potassium, Magnesium, and Heart Disease[1]

Although hypertension is a circulatory problem, it is usually caused by renal rather than heart disease in dogs and cats. The renal causes and their management are described in Chapter 13. Feeding low-sodium diets is an important part of management (see Table 16.1 for sodium contents of foods). Because renal disease impairs all kidney functions, dietary intake of other salts must also be restricted. Recipes for this management are found in Chapter 13.

Congestive heart failure develops when the heart no longer sustains normal circulation. Compensatory mechanisms attempt to restore normal circulation. The mechanisms attempt to maintain blood pressure, fluid volume, sodium concentration, delivery of oxygen and nutrients, removal of carbon dioxide and other waste products, as well as delivery of regulating agents and hormones. Circulating blood volume depends on total body sodium, which determines extracellular fluid.

Table 16.1. Sodium content of foods (milligrams sodium/110 grams food)

Foods from plants	Mg sodium	Foods from animals	Mg sodium
Barley (pearled)	3	Beef hamburger	200
Rice (white)	3	Beef chuck	104
Farina	2	Chicken, light meat	190
Wheat	2	Chicken, dark meat	255
Oatmeal	5	Cottage cheese	1055
Baked breads	500–1000	Egg yolk	51
Potatoes (sweet)	28	Egg, whole	311
Corn flakes	1045	Beef kidney	730
Crackers	1100	Beef liver	453
Pretzels	1361	Beef heart	382
Squash	Trace	Bacon and ham	1100–1800
Soybean (tofu)	7	Frankfurter	2477
Cornmeal	1	Cheese (processed)	1890
Potatoes (white)	5	Canned beef stew	2349

Source: Morris (1995).

Regulation to maintain normal body sodium is lost with congestive heart failure and also with some heart diseases that are not causing clinical signs. Renal sodium excretion is reduced below normal, and sodium is retained, resulting in water retention. Clinical signs are not apparent in early cases. Ascites and edema appear in severe retention. Pulmonary edema can develop and cause respiratory failure.

Sodium retention is managed by feeding a low-sodium diet, beginning before signs of congestive heart failure appear. Low-sodium diets are usually effective. Sodium content of different foods are shown in Table 16.1. When dietary management begins after clinical signs appear, improvement may not be evident without other treatment such as diuretics. Diuretics can cause loss of enough sodium to produce hyponatremia, which can result in neurological signs. In recently developed cases a low-sodium diet should be tried first, and diuretics should be used only when dietary management alone fails.

Potassium depletion is common in patients with heart disease. Potassium deficiency follows because poor appetite reduces intake, and diuretics, hyperaldosteronism, and persistent chloride depletion increase renal loss. Very low sodium diets stimulate aldosterone release to conserve sodium, but aldosterone stimulates renal potassium excretion. Potassium losses are reflected by hypokalemia, but they can be predicted even when plasma potassium levels are normal. Hypokalemia increases toxicity to drugs such as cardiac glycosides. Also, hypokalemia reduces efficacy of some antiarrhythmic drugs. Unless plasma electrolyte measurements show hyperkalemia, animals with heart disease should receive dietary levels of potassium higher than what the National Research Council recommends.

Magnesium depletion is often unrecognized in animals with heart disease. The causes include reduced intake and increased renal loss due to diuretics or chronic use of other drugs that promote renal magnesium excretion. Cardiac glycosides promote renal wasting of magnesium. Magnesium, like potassium, is largely intracellular. Plasma magnesium concentrations account for only 1 percent of total magnesium and do not reflect body stores. Magnesium depletion is difficult to prove by plasma levels. Muscle biopsy magnesium measurements reliably reflect total body amounts. Low plasma magnesium during cardiac glycoside and diuretic therapy justifies magnesium replacement therapy.

Cardiac Cachexia[1]

Cardiac cachexia is the loss of body fat and skeletal muscle with chronic congestive heart failure. Its causes include reduced appetite, poorer assimilation of food, increased energy expenditure, and drugs for treating heart disease and its complications.

Animals with chronic congestive heart failure often become anorectic for reasons poorly understood. Anorexia is worsened by unpalatable diets: severe sodium and protein restriction can reduce food intake.

Appetite can be normal, but malabsorption of nutrients can be great enough to cause weight loss. Congestive heart failure causes hypertension in intestinal capillaries, veins, and lymphatics. In addition to reducing nutrient absorption, hypertension causes plasma and lymph fluid loss into the intestine. This protein-losing enteropathy results in protein depletion as well as the loss of other substances in plasma.

Metabolic rates increase with chronic congestive heart failure. Increased energy is needed to support greater efforts to sustain respiration and circulation.

Drugs commonly used to manage chronic congestive heart failure, such as cardiac glycosides, can reduce appetite, cause vomiting, and impair intestinal absorption. Diuretics can cause electrolyte imbalances, which can affect appetite and intestinal absorption.

Diets for Dogs and Cats with Chronic Heart Disease[1]

Diets for management of heart disease must contain normal amounts of taurine and L-carnitine. Beef-based diets provide more L-carnitine than chicken-based diets. Both beef and chicken provide taurine. Sodium-restricted diets must be used for animals with sodium and fluid retention, hypertension, or congestive heart failure. Potassium supplementation is necessary with suspected or proven potassium depletion. With increased plasma potassium, dietary potassium should be low. Magnesium is often lost, so dietary magnesium should be higher than usual. Diets should be highly palatable. Vitamin B_{12} should be given by tablet several times a month or by feeding a food such as sardines that contains abundant amounts.

■ Diets for Chronic Heart Disease in Dogs

Beef, Potato, and Chicken Fat Diet (Normal protein, high-potassium, minimum sodium, high-fat)

8 ounces lean ground beef (raw weight), cooked

3 cups potato, boiled with skin

1 tablespoon chicken fat

5 bonemeal tablets (10-grain or equivalent)

1 multiple vitamin-mineral tablet

Provides 909 kilocalories, 47.8 grams protein, 37.9 grams fat
Supports caloric needs of a 31-pound dog
Provides sodium at 105 percent, potassium at 254 percent, magnesium at 212 percent of a dog's daily needs

---

Beef and Potato Diet (Normal protein, high-potassium, minimum sodium, moderate fat)

8 ounces lean ground beef (raw weight), cooked

3 cups potato, boiled with skin

5 bonemeal tablets (10-grain or equivalent)

1 multiple vitamin-mineral tablet

Provides 792 kilocalories, 47.8 grams protein, 24.9 grams fat
Supports caloric needs of a 26-pound dog
Provides sodium at 112 percent, potassium at 262 percent, magnesium at 229 percent of a dog's daily needs

Chicken, Potato, and Chicken Fat Diet (Normal protein, high-potassium, minimum sodium, moderate fat)

1 cup cooked chicken breast

3 cups potato, boiled with skin

1 tablespoon chicken fat

5 bonemeal tablets (10-grain or equivalent)

1 multiple vitamin-mineral tablet

Provides 735 kilocalories, 49.7 grams protein, 17.8 grams fat
Supports caloric needs of a 23- to 24-pound dog
Provides sodium at 108 percent, potassium at 261 percent, magnesium at 244 percent of a dog's daily needs

Chicken and Potato Diet (Normal protein, high-potassium, minimum sodium, low-fat)

1 cup cooked chicken breast

3 cups potato, boiled with skin

4 bonemeal tablets (10-grain or equivalent)

1 multiple vitamin-mineral tablet

Provides 620 kilocalories, 49.7 grams protein, 4.8 grams fat
Supports caloric needs of a 23- to 24-pound dog
Provides sodium at 119 percent, potassium at 287 percent, magnesium at 262 percent of a dog's daily needs

Beef, Rice, and Chicken Fat Diet (Normal protein, low-potassium, minimum sodium, high-fat)

8 ounces lean ground beef (raw weight), cooked

2 cups rice, long-grain, cooked

1 tablespoon chicken fat

5 bonemeal tablets (10-grain or equivalent)

1 multiple vitamin-mineral tablet

Provides 913 kilocalories, 47.6 grams protein, 38.1 grams fat
Supports caloric needs of a 31-pound dog
Provides sodium at 98 percent, potassium at 61 percent, magnesium at 135 percent of a dog's daily needs
Add salt substitute (potassium chloride, 1/4 teaspoon) to bring potassium to 137 percent of needs.

Beef and Rice Diet (Normal protein, low-potassium, minimum sodium, moderate fat)

8 ounces lean ground beef (raw weight), cooked

2 cups rice, long-grain, cooked

4 bonemeal tablets (10-grain or equivalent)

1 multiple vitamin-mineral tablet

Provides 796 kilocalories, 47.6 grams protein, 25.3 grams fat
Supports caloric needs of a 26-pound dog
Provides sodium at 101 percent, potassium at 65 percent, magnesium at 146 percent of a dog's daily needs
Add salt substitute (potassium chloride, 1/4 teaspoon) to bring potassium to 147 percent of needs.

Chicken, Rice, and Chicken Fat Diet (Normal protein, low-potassium, minimum sodium, moderate fat)

1 cup cooked chicken breast

2 cups rice, long-grain, cooked

1 tablespoon chicken fat

4 bonemeal tablets (10-grain or equivalent)

1 multiple vitamin-mineral tablet

Provides 739 kilocalories, 49.5 grams protein, 18 grams fat
Supports caloric needs of a 23- to 24-pound dog
Provides sodium at 103 percent, potassium at 65 percent, magnesium at 159 percent of a dog's daily needs
Add salt substitute (potassium chloride, ¼ teaspoon) to bring potassium to 136 percent of needs.

Chicken and Rice Diet (Normal protein, low-potassium, minimum sodium, low-fat)

1 cup cooked chicken breast

2 cups rice, long-grain, cooked

4 bonemeal tablets (10-grain or equivalent)

1 multiple vitamin-mineral tablet

Provides 624 kilocalories, 49.5 grams protein, 5.25 grams fat
Supports caloric needs of a 26-pound dog
Provides sodium at 103 percent, potassium at 56 percent, magnesium at 173 percent of a dog's daily needs
Add salt substitute (potassium chloride, ¼ teaspoon) to bring potassium to 147 percent of needs.

■ Diets for Chronic Heart Disease in Cats

Beef, Rice, Clams, and Chicken Fat Diet (Normal protein, normal potassium, minimum sodium)

8 ounces lean ground beef (raw weight), cooked

½ cup rice, long-grain, cooked

1 ounce clams, chopped in juice

½ tablespoon chicken fat

2 bonemeal tablets (10-grain or equivalent)

½ calcium carbonate tablet (200 milligrams calcium)

1 multiple vitamin-mineral tablet

Provides 590 kilocalories, 48.7 grams protein, 31.6 grams fat
Use Table 4.4 in Chapter 4 to determine how much to feed.
Provides potassium at 164 percent, sodium at 276 percent, magnesium at 167 percent of a cat's daily needs

---

Beef, Clams, and Chicken Fat Diet (Normal protein, normal potassium, moderate sodium)

8 ounces lean ground beef (raw weight), cooked

1 ounce clams, chopped in juice

½ tablespoon chicken fat

1 bonemeal tablet (10-grain or equivalent)

1 calcium carbonate tablet (400 milligrams calcium)

1 multiple vitamin-mineral tablet

Provides 487 kilocalories, 46.6 grams protein, 31.4 grams fat
Use Table 4.4 in Chapter 4 to determine how much to feed.
Provides potassium at 202 percent, sodium at 362 percent, magnesium at 174 percent of a cat's daily needs

Chicken, Rice, Clams, and Chicken Fat Diet (Normal protein, normal potassium, moderate sodium)

1 cup cooked chicken breast

½ cup rice, long-grain, cooked

1 ounce clams, chopped in juice

1 tablespoon chicken fat

1 bonemeal tablet (10-grain or equivalent)

1 calcium carbonate tablet (400 milligrams calcium)

1 multiple vitamin-mineral tablet

Provides 475 kilocalories, 50.2 grams protein, 18.1 grams fat
Use Table 4.4 in Chapter 4 to determine how much to feed.
Provides potassium at 150 percent, sodium at 308 percent, magnesium at 203 percent of a cat's daily needs

Chicken, Clams, and Chicken Fat Diet (Normal protein, normal potassium, moderate sodium)

1 cup cooked chicken breast

1 ounce clams, chopped in juice

1 tablespoon chicken fat

1 bonemeal tablet (10-grain or equivalent)

1 calcium carbonate tablet (400 milligrams calcium)

1 multiple vitamin-mineral tablet

Provides 372 kilocalories, 48.1 grams protein, 17.9 grams fat
Use Table 4.4 in Chapter 4 to determine how much to feed.
Provides potassium at 189 percent, sodium at 409 percent, magnesium at 232 percent of a cat's daily needs

Tuna, Clams, and Rice Diet (*Normal protein, normal potassium, minimum sodium*)

5½ ounces tuna, canned in water (low-sodium)

1 ounce clams, chopped in juice

½ cup rice, long-grain, cooked

1 tablespoon chicken fat

1 bonemeal tablet (10-grain or equivalent)

1 calcium carbonate tablet (400 milligrams calcium)

1 multiple vitamin-mineral tablet

Provides 431 kilocalories, 46.4 grams protein, 16.6 grams fat
Use Table 4.4 in Chapter 4 to determine how much to feed.
Provides potassium at 149 percent and magnesium at 605 percent of a cat's daily needs. Sodium is low depending on content in tuna fish.

Tuna and Clams Diet (*Normal protein, normal potassium, minimum sodium*)

5½ ounces tuna, canned in water (low-sodium)

1 ounce clams, chopped in juice

1 tablespoon chicken fat

1 calcium carbonate tablet (400 milligrams calcium)

1 multiple vitamin-mineral tablet

Provides 328 kilocalories, 44.3 grams protein, 16.4 grams fat
Use Table 4.4 in Chapter 4 to determine how much to feed.
Provides potassium at 200 percent and magnesium at 808 percent of a cat's daily needs. Sodium is low depending on content in tuna fish.

Reference

1. Stepien, Rebecca L. and Matthew W. Miller. 1994. Cardiovascular disease. In *The Waltham Book of Clinical Nutrition of the Dog and Cat*, edited by J.M. Wills and K.W. Simpson, 353–371. Oxford: Pergamon Press.

2. Morris, James G. 1995. *Nutrition and Nutritional Diseases in Animals*. 10-1 to 10-27. Class Notes for Veterinary Medicine 408, School of Veterinary Medicine, University of California, Davis.

CHAPTER 17
Diet and Pancreatic Disease

A pancreatic disease that both dogs and cats develop is pancreatitis, where inflammation destroys part or all of the tissue that produces digestive enzymes. Pancreatic enzyme insufficiency, another pancreatic disease, appears in certain breeds of dogs and is thought to be a congenital defect. Insufficiency can also develop from inflammation destroying secretory tissue. An important treatment for both diseases is dietary. Pancreatic tumors are relatively uncommon in dogs and cats and cannot be managed by diet.

Pancreatitis

■ Etiology and Pathogenesis[1]

Pancreatic inflammation is relatively common and sometimes life threatening. Most cases (about two-thirds) of pancreatitis are secondary to a problem in another organ or tissue. Secondary causes include renal, gastrointestinal, hepatic, and cardiovascular disease. Cancer in the pancreas or other organs, generalized infections, and drugs can also cause pancreatitis. Primary pancreatitis represents the remaining third of cases.

The cause of primary pancreatitis is unknown. Acute primary pancreatitis has been thought to be caused by what an animal eats. Many have a history of eating high-fat meals or table scraps in garbage. High-fat meals are thought to be a significant cause of acute pancreatitis. However, high-fat meals are routinely fed to some working dogs with no ill effects. Sled dogs can live on a diet containing 60 percent fat and have no problems. Despite that, very low fat diets are fed during and after recovery from acute pancreatitis.

Foods with the greatest potential for stimulating pancreatic enzyme secretion are believed to cause pancreatitis. Protein and fat are the most potent stimulators. During recovery from acute pancreatitis, animals are often fed high-carbohydrate, low-fat, and low-protein diets. Animals with abundant pancreatic stores of digestive enzymes are most susceptible to acute pancreatitis. Undernourished animals are less likely to develop pancreatitis when they are fed a diet rich in protein and fat. Feeding a diet deficient in some important nutrients can cause pancreatitis, however. A deficiency of choline and methionine destabilizes pancreatic membranes, isolating pancreatic enzymes before they are secreted. Membrane instability causes enzymes to leak into pancreatic tissue and leads to inflammation and necrosis.

Overweight and overnourished animals are more likely to develop acute pancreatitis. Obese middle-aged dogs are at highest risk for pancreatitis. They have rich stores of pancreatic enzymes and are the most likely to eat foods rich in protein and fat. Management to reduce the risk of pancreatitis must include maintaining body weight within normal limits.

Dietary constituents other than nutrients contribute to acute pancreatitis. Bacteria and other infectious agents can cause pancreatitis. Bacteria are common in many commercial dry pet foods, and their numbers can increase after food is moistened. Bacteria can reflux from the intestine through the pancreatic duct and into the pancreas. They can also cross the intestinal wall and enter the pancreas, lying adjacent. Animals with acute pancreatitis have bacteremia and bacteria in the pancreas. Regardless of whether this is a primary or secondary phenomenon, affected animals must be treated with antibiotics.

Commercial pet foods and foods contaminated by coliform bacteria contain endotoxin. Their consumption can result in endotoxemia. Endotoxemia is a feature of acute pancreatitis and contributes to the damage, partly because endotoxin disrupts pancreatic microcirculation.

Pancreatitis can be produced by allergic or immune-mediated reactions. If such reactions are against dietary antigens, controlled diets would reduce relapses and hasten recovery.

■ Diagnosis[1]

Acute pancreatitis is often difficult to diagnose. In dogs usual clinical signs are vomiting, anorexia, and abdominal pain. In some cases none of these signs may be seen, which may make it seem that acute pancreatitis is unlikely. Other signs include depression, fever, diarrhea, abdominal distention, dehydration and shock, respiratory distress, and cardiac arrhythmias. Often the only signs are anorexia and depression.

Chronic pancreatitis in dogs and cats is difficult to recognize because they usually show no clinical signs. In some dogs chronic pancreatitis causes diabetes mellitus, but signs of pancreatitis were never seen when inflammation destroyed the pancreas.

Cats with acute pancreatitis show fewer diagnostic signs than dogs. Most cats are never diagnosed with pancreatitis until necropsy because no signs are evident to suspect pancreatitis.

Acute pancreatitis is proven in dogs by identifying increased plasma lipase activity. No other clinical pathology tests, such as for plasma amylase activity, are reliable in identifying acute pancreatitis. Not all animals with increased plasma lipase activity have pancreatitis. About 75 percent have pancreatitis, with the other 25 percent having a problem such as renal, hepatic, or neoplastic disease.

Abdominal ultrasound is used to confirm that increased plasma lipase activity is due to pancreatitis and not due to another problem. The normal pancreas is not seen with ultrasound, but inflammation causes it to be visible. Other diagnostic studies, such as abdominal radiography, can be done, but they either are unreliable or provide no additional useful information.

Plasma lipase activity is usually normal in dogs with chronic pancreatitis. Abdominal ultrasound is the only diagnostic tool useful for the identification of chronic pancreatitis. The chronically diseased pancreas is visible on ultrasound.

Plasma lipase activity increases in cats with acute pancreatitis, but it returns to normal in four to five days. Ultrasound is useful in identifying cats with acute pancreatitis.

■ Management[1]

Medical Treatment
Intravenous fluids and antibiotics are essential in treating dogs and cats with acute pancreatitis. Without fluid therapy mortality can be high. Many other treatments are described, but none are of any proven value. During the initial acute phase, no food is given. Many animals are anorectic and vomiting, so offering food is of no value. Food is avoided because feeding stimulates the pancreas to secrete, which is thought to worsen its inflammation.

Dietary Treatment

Feeding can begin for dogs four to five days after the onset of acute pancreatitis. Carbohydrates and electrolytes are given first; they stimulate pancreatic secretion little. Initial feedings can be glucose solutions, and gradually an easily digested starch such as boiled rice can be given. Proteins of high biological value, such as egg white, are added next. Whole eggs are not fed because their yolks are high in fat. Other low-fat proteins with high biological value include low-fat cottage cheese and lean meat such as chicken breast. Vitamin B_{12} should be given by tablet several times a month or by feeding a food such as sardines that contains abundant amounts.

Recovering cats are fed following the principles for dogs. Cats have a higher protein requirement, and they are not likely to accept the same foods as dogs. Cats should also be fed a relatively low-fat diet. However, no one has shown that cats recover poorly if they are fed a high-fat diet.

If pancreatitis results from an immune-mediated or allergic response to something in the diet, a controlled diet must be fed.

■ Diets for Dogs with Pancreatitis

Cottage Cheese and Rice Diet (Low-fat, low-protein)

½ cup cottage cheese, 1 percent fat

2 cups rice, long-grain, cooked

Egg yolk of 1 egg, large, hard-boiled

3 bonemeal tablets (10-grain or equivalent)

¼ teaspoon salt substitute—potassium chloride

1 multiple vitamin-mineral tablet

Provides 551 kilocalories, 25.4 grams protein, 7.2 grams fat
Supports caloric needs of a 16-pound dog
Choline content is higher than with vegetable oil.

Cottage Cheese and Rice Diet (*Low-fat, low-protein*)

½ *cup cottage cheese, 1 percent fat*

2 cups rice, long-grain, cooked

1 teaspoon vegetable (canola) oil

3 bonemeal tablets (10-grain or equivalent)

¼ *teaspoon salt substitute—potassium chloride*

multiple vitamin-mineral tablet

Provides 535 kilocalories, 22.6 grams protein, 6.9 grams fat
Supports caloric needs of a 15-pound dog

Egg Whites and Rice Diet (*Low-fat, low-protein*)

Egg whites of 4 eggs, large, hard-boiled

2 cups rice, long-grain, cooked

Egg yolk of 1 egg, large, hard-boiled

3 bonemeal tablets (10-grain or equivalent)

¼ *teaspoon salt substitute—potassium chloride*

1 multiple vitamin-mineral tablet

Provides 537 kilocalories, 25.4 grams protein, 6.1 grams fat
Supports caloric needs of a 16-pound dog
Choline content is higher than with vegetable oil.

Egg Whites and Rice Diet (Low-fat, low-protein)

Egg whites of 4 eggs, large, hard-boiled

Egg yolks of 2 eggs, large, hard-boiled

2 cups rice, long-grain, cooked

3 bonemeal tablets (10-grain or equivalent)

¼ teaspoon salt substitute—potassium chloride

⅕ multiple vitamin-mineral tablet

Provides 597 kilocalories, 28.2 grams protein, 11.2 grams fat
Supports caloric needs of an 18-pound dog
Choline content is higher than with vegetable oil.

Egg Whites and Rice Diet (Low-fat, low-protein)

Egg whites of 4 eggs, large, hard-boiled

2 cups rice, long-grain, cooked

1 teaspoon vegetable (canola) oil

4 bonemeal tablets (10-grain or equivalent)

¼ teaspoon salt substitute—potassium chloride

1 multiple vitamin-mineral tablet

Provides 520 kilocalories, 22.4 grams protein, 5.8 grams fat
Supports caloric needs of a 14- to 15-pound dog
Choline content is lower with vegetable oil.

Egg Whites and Rice Diet (Low-fat, low-protein)

Egg whites of 4 eggs, large, hard-boiled

2 cups rice, long-grain, cooked

2 teaspoons vegetable (canola) oil

4 bonemeal tablets (10-grain or equivalent)

¼ teaspoon salt substitute—potassium chloride

1 multiple vitamin-mineral tablet

Provides 561 kilocalories, 22.4 grams protein, 10.4 grams fat
Supports caloric needs of a 16-pound dog
Choline content is lower with vegetable oil.

Chicken and Rice Diet (Low-fat, low-protein)

½ cup chicken breast, cooked

2 cups rice, long-grain, cooked

1 teaspoon vegetable (canola) oil

4 bonemeal tablets (10-grain or equivalent)

⅒ teaspoon table salt

¼ teaspoon salt substitute—potassium chloride

1 multiple vitamin-mineral tablet

Provides 562 kilocalories, 28.9 grams protein, 7.8 grams fat
Supports caloric needs of a 16-pound dog
Choline content is lower with vegetable oil.

Chicken and Rice Diet (*Low-fat, low-protein*)

$1/2$ *cup chicken breast, cooked*

Egg yolk of 1 egg, large, hard-boiled

2 cups rice, long-grain, cooked

3 bonemeal tablets (10-grain or equivalent)

$1/10$ *teaspoon table salt*

$1/4$ *teaspoon salt substitute—potassium chloride*

1 multiple vitamin-mineral tablet

Provides 577 kilocalories, 31.8 grams protein, 8.2 grams fat
Supports caloric needs of a 17-pound dog
Choline content is higher with egg yolk.

Chicken and Potato Diet (*Low-fat, moderate protein*)

1 cup chicken breast, cooked

3 cups potato, cooked with skin

1 teaspoon vegetable (canola) oil

4 bonemeal tablets (10-grain or equivalent)

1 multiple vitamin-mineral tablet

Provides 662 kilocalories, 49.4 grams protein, 9.4 grams fat
Supports caloric needs of a 20-pound dog

Chicken and Potato Diet (Very low fat, moderate protein)

1 cup chicken breast, cooked

3 cups potato, cooked with skin

4 bonemeal tablets (10-grain or equivalent)

1 multiple vitamin-mineral tablet

Provides 622 kilocalories, 49.5 grams protein, 4.9 grams fat
Supports caloric needs of an 18- to 19-pound dog

Cottage Cheese and Potato Diet (Low-fat, moderate protein)

1 cup cottage cheese, 1 percent fat

3 cups potato, cooked with skin

1 teaspoon vegetable (canola) oil

4 bonemeal tablets (10-grain or equivalent)

1 multiple vitamin-mineral tablet

Provides 615 kilocalories, 36.8 grams protein, 7.6 grams fat
Supports caloric needs of an 18-pound dog

Cottage Cheese and Potato Diet (Very low fat, moderate protein)

1 cup cottage cheese, 1 percent fat

3 cups potato, cooked with skin

3 bonemeal tablets (10-grain or equivalent)

1 multiple vitamin-mineral tablet

Provides 574 kilocalories, 36.8 grams protein, 3 grams fat
Supports caloric needs of a 17-pound dog

Egg Whites and Potato Diet (Low-fat, low-protein)

Egg whites of 4 eggs, large, hard-boiled

2 cups potato, cooked with skin

1 teaspoon vegetable (canola) oil

3 bonemeal tablets (10-grain or equivalent)

1 multiple vitamin-mineral tablet

Provides 381 kilocalories, 19.8 grams protein, 5.1 grams fat
Supports caloric needs of a 9- to 10-pound dog

Egg Whites and Potato Diet (Low-fat, low-protein)

Egg whites of 4 eggs, large, hard-boiled

2 cups potato, cooked with skin

Egg yolk of 1 egg, large, hard-boiled

3 bonemeal tablets (10-grain or equivalent)

1 multiple vitamin-mineral tablet

Provides 397 kilocalories, 22.7 grams protein, 5.4 grams fat
Supports caloric needs of a 10- to 11-pound dog
Choline content is higher with egg yolk.

Pancreatic Enzyme Insufficiency[1,2]

Chronic relapsing pancreatitis and juvenile pancreatic atrophy are the most common causes of deficient pancreatic secretion. The latter appears in young dogs, with German shepherds most commonly affected, suggesting the problem is congenital in that breed. Clinical signs frequently do not appear until the animal is 6 to 12 months old, which suggests that enzyme secretion is adequate in very early life. Other possible causes include viral infection and abnormal immune-mediated damage to pancreatic acinar tissue.

Clinical signs of pancreatic insufficiency in dogs are weight loss, bulky feces that can be formed or loose, and increased appetite. Feces show steatorrhea and other signs of undigested food. Steatorrhea is most easily confirmed by fecal smears stained with Sudan stain to show fat globules. Steatorrhea also results from many other causes of maldigestion and malabsorption, so pancreatic enzyme insufficiency must be confirmed with another test. Measurement of serum trypsin-like immunoreactivity is used to confirm a diagnosis.

Pancreatic enzyme insufficiency is most importantly treated with pancreatic enzymes in the form of a powder mixed with food. Digestion is more complete, and less enzyme-replacement therapy is needed when an owner-prepared, rather than commercial, pet food is fed. The diet should be made with foods having the highest digestibility and should be low in fiber to maximize digestibility. Excess carbohydrates should be avoided because they escape optimum digestion, even with enzymes added to the diet. Still, increased calories are needed to restore weight losses. It may be best to accomplish that with fat rather than carbohydrates. A readily digested protein is fed. Affected dogs should be fed three times a day. The following recipes include low-fat and moderate to high-fat diets. Dogs may respond to one type better than the other. Use the diet that gives the best results in restoring weight loss and producing normal feces.

■ **Diets for Pancreatic Enzyme Insufficiency**

Cottage Cheese and Boiled Rice Diet (Low-fat)

⅔ *cup cottage cheese, 1 percent fat*

2 cups rice, long-grain, cooked

1 teaspoon vegetable oil

¼ teaspoon salt substitute—potassium chloride

3 bonemeal tablets (10-grain or equivalent)

1 multiple vitamin-mineral tablet

Provides 564 kilocalories, 27.1 grams protein, 7.4 grams fat
Supports caloric needs of a 16- to 17-pound dog

Chicken and Rice Diet (Low-fat)

$\frac{1}{2}$ cup chicken breast, cooked

2 cups rice, long-grain, cooked

Egg yolk of 1 egg, large, hard-boiled

3 bonemeal tablets (10-grain or equivalent)

$\frac{1}{10}$ teaspoon table salt

$\frac{1}{4}$ teaspoon salt substitute—potassium chloride

1 multiple vitamin-mineral tablet

Provides 577 kilocalories, 31.8 grams protein, 8.2 grams fat
Supports caloric needs of a 17-pound dog

Cottage Cheese and Rice Diet (Moderate to high-fat)

1 cup cottage cheese, 2 percent fat

$2\frac{1}{2}$ cups rice, long-grain, cooked

2 tablespoons sardines, canned, tomato sauce

$1\frac{1}{2}$ tablespoons vegetable (canola) oil

$\frac{1}{4}$ teaspoon salt substitute—potassium chloride

4 bonemeal tablets (10-grain or equivalent)

1 multiple vitamin-mineral tablet

Provides 973 kilocalories, 47.8 grams protein, 31.2 grams fat
Supports caloric needs of a 34-pound dog
Omission of sardines reduces caloric content by 68 kilocalories, protein by 6.2 grams, and fat by 4.6 grams.

Poultry Meat and Potato Diet (*Moderate to high-fat*)

⅓ *pound poultry meat (raw weight), cooked*

2 *tablespoons sardines, canned, tomato sauce*

3 *cups potato, cooked with skin*

1 *tablespoon vegetable (canola) oil*

¼ *teaspoon salt substitute—potassium chloride*

¹⁄₁₀ *teaspoon table salt*

4 *bonemeal tablets (10-grain or equivalent)*

1 *multiple vitamin-mineral tablet*

Provides 851 kilocalories, 42.4 grams protein, 34.3 grams fat
Supports caloric needs of a 28- to 29-pound dog
Omission of sardines reduces caloric content by 68 kilocalories, protein by 6.2 grams, and fat by 4.6 grams.

References

1. Williams, David A. 1996. Malabsorption, small intestinal bacterial overgrowth, and protein-losing enteropathy. In *Strombeck's Small Animal Gastroenterology*, edited by W. Grant Guilford, Sharon A. Center, Donald R. Strombeck, David A. Williams, and Denny J. Meyer, 381–410. Philadelphia: W.B. Saunders.

2. Williams, David A. 1996. The pancreas. In *Strombeck's Small Animal Gastroenterology*, edited by W. Grant Guilford, Sharon A. Center, Donald R. Strombeck, David A. Williams, and Denny J. Meyer, 367–380. Philadelphia: W.B. Saunders.

CHAPTER 18
Diet and Hepatic Disease

Hepatic disease is common in dogs and cats. Few cases were recognized 30 years ago. With current diagnostic procedures it is possible to identify nearly all cases of hepatic disease early so treatment can be successful. The liver is damaged by many injuries and diseases elsewhere in the body. Thus, many different diseases need management to protect and heal the liver. Hepatic disease also develops that is unrelated to pathology outside the liver.

A variety of toxins damage the liver. They include drugs, chemicals, and microbial toxins. Often drugs must be discontinued before the liver can recover. Most toxic chemicals enter orally, with their primary source being food. Commercial pet foods contain chemicals that can be changed by intestinal bacteria to hepatotoxins. Pet foods also contain endotoxin, produced from bacteria, which can damage the liver. Many commercial pet foods contain little endotoxin while others contain large amounts. Endotoxin is often not injurious unless another chemical, such as a drug, is present. A synergistic action of the two causes liver damage (see Chapter 3).

Commercial pet foods seldom contain substances that cause primary hepatic disease in an animal, but their composition can interfere with its recovery. Pet food companies prepare no products for treating hepatic disease. They often recommend products for treating renal disease because these are low-protein diets. Treatment of hepatic disease requires more, however. Feeding a special, owner-prepared diet is essential for managing hepatic disease and is more important than any other treatment.

Very few forms of hepatic disease need drugs for recovery. As mentioned, most cases should be given no drugs because the liver must metabolize many drugs for excretion, a function that is often reduced by disease.

Evaluation of Dogs and Cats for Hepatic Disease[1,2]

Dogs and cats show few clinical signs with early hepatic disease. They include anorexia, depression, and often increased water consumption. Unfortunately, these signs are common with many problems, and no clinical signs are specific for hepatic disease. Hepatic disease is possible with any unexplained clinical signs. On waiting for these signs to disappear spontaneously, many cases of hepatic disease worsen. Hepatic disease can be difficult to treat when it is not recognized early.

No physical findings are pathognomonic for hepatic disease. Findings such as jaundice or ascites more commonly indicate nonhepatic problems.

Blood-screening tests help evaluate unexplained clinical findings caused by hepatic disease. One evaluates alanine aminotransferase (ALT) enzyme activity, which is restricted to liver cells. With damage ALT leaks out, and its plasma activity increases. Other blood chemistry tests are not specific for hepatic injury.

Reduced appetite is the earliest sign of hepatic disease. Other signs subsequently appear with worsening disease and loss of hepatic function. They include depression, weakness, and signs of hepatic encephalopathy. The most important cause of encephalopathy is increased blood ammonia. The normal liver removes ammonia and converts it to urea; ammonia is toxic and urea is not. Ammonia tolerance testing can be done to evaluate this function. No other test is reliable for determining whether hepatic disease is responsible for loss of appetite or any other signs.

Although other tests can be done to evaluate for hepatic disease, most do not provide useful information. For example, radiographs of the liver are almost never valuable in identifying hepatic disease.

Liver biopsy is always useful in evaluating for liver damage, but in many cases liver biopsy is not necessary because disease outside the liver is responsible for hepatic damage. Once a nonhepatic problem is recognized and understood, liver biopsy is often not needed because any secondary hepatic pathology is predictable and does not need to be proven with a biopsy. However, with primary hepatic disease a liver biopsy is important for treatment and prognosis.

Management of Hepatic Disease[1-6]

Dogs and cats with hepatic disease and hepatic insufficiency should always be treated dietarily. Special consideration should usually be given to caloric intake, carbohydrate quantity and quality, protein quantity and quality, fat quantity and quality, sodium restriction, potassium supplementation, and supplementation or restriction of vitamins and micronutrients. In addition, management may be necessary for hepatic encephalopathy, hepatic inflammation and fibrosis, toxins absorbed from the intestine, infection, fluid retention, altered drug metabolism, retention of bile acids, and complications such as gastric ulceration and hemorrhage. Portasystemic shunts are also managed surgically.

An initial goal in managing dogs and cats with hepatic insufficiency is to reduce intestinal toxin production and absorption. Such management includes defined-protein diets, antibiotics to reduce intestinal bacteria, and cathartics to minimize toxin absorption. Medical treatment for hepatic encephalopathy is generally unsuccessful.

Feeding is essential for management of hepatic disease. No drug helps recovery from hepatic damage; only feeding assists recovery. With anorexia there is no chance for recovery, and hepatic damage worsens. Fasting depletes glutathione and other nutrients needed to protect hepatocytes and to reduce further damage. Energy and a balanced supply of nutrients are needed for arresting degeneration and supporting hepatic regeneration.

Diets for Dogs and Cats with Hepatic Disease

■ Carbohydrates

Dietary carbohydrates should be high-quality and highly digestible. Bacteria ferment undigested carbohydrates entering the colon. Such fermentation increases colonic bacteria that degrade proteins and urea to form ammonia. The colon absorbs ammonia, and blood ammonia increases.

Carbohydrates minimize amino acid catabolism for energy, especially catabolism of the branched-chain amino acids, which are used for energy and found at reduced levels. High dietary carbohydrate promotes insulin secretion and reduced glucagon release. That ratio favors anabolic conditions where amino acids absorbed from the intestine are converted to protein rather than metabolized to glucose. Catabolic conditions produce ammonia.

Dietary carbohydrates are increased during management of episodic hypoglycemia and ammonia intolerance. Frequent feedings of simple and complex carbohydrates are of benefit. Simple and complex carbohydrates are provided by boiled white rice, potatoes, and vegetables. Simple carbohydrates are nearly completely digested and absorbed. Vegetables provide complex carbohydrates as fiber. Fiber reduces availability and absorption of such toxins as endotoxin, other bacterial toxins, and some bile acids. Fiber also promotes fecal excretion of ammonia, so less is absorbed. Fiber slows dietary carbohydrate absorption, which maintains normal blood glucose in patients intermittently hypoglycemic and hyperglycemic.

■ Proteins

Dietary proteins can be reduced but only with signs of protein intolerance. Hepatic regeneration requires maintained protein intake; protein requirements are greater during recovering from hepatic disease. In general, feed as much protein as can be tolerated. Giving too much causes hepatic encephalopathy to appear or worsen.

Ammonia Intoxication

Ammonia is probably the most important toxin absorbed from the intestine. Approximately one-half is derived from bacterial activity and the other half from glutamine metabolism. The colon produces most ammonia from bacterial activity.

Intestinal bacteria produce ammonia by urease activity or by deaminating peptides. Urea diffuses from extracellular fluid into the intestine in amounts determined by dietary nitrogen levels. Dietary levels and kinds of protein and any unusual loss of blood or plasma protein into the intestine determine colonic peptide levels. With appropriate dietary protein, digestion and absorption are optimal, so little dietary nitrogen enters the colon.

Protein also enters the colon in desquamated mucosal cells and plasma proteins. Desquamation of small intestinal mucosa is minimal when intestinal contents are scanty. Low-roughage diets minimize desquamation. Protein-losing enteropathy can cause entry of excess plasma proteins into the colon. Hypoproteinemia is most commonly caused by protein-losing enteropathy and infrequently caused by hepatic disease impairing protein synthesis.

Protein Restriction

Because hyperammonemia causes the earliest and most important signs of hepatic disease, treatment is sometimes necessary to reduce blood ammonia. Because all ammonia comes directly or indirectly from dietary protein, hepatic disease is often managed with low-protein diets. Adequate protein is needed to restore normal hepatic structure and function, however. The liver also produces and exports proteins such as for plasma. Reducing protein intake can compromise hepatic function so the liver cannot recover. Proper management of hepatic disease includes feeding as much protein as can be tolerated. Greater success is evident when only high-quality proteins are fed. Proteins with high biological value are used completely, leaving little for conversion to ammonia. Commercial pet foods contain little high-quality protein, so they are not useful for managing hepatic disease. The following diets contain only high-quality proteins.

When little or no protein is given and calories are supplied by glucose, nitrogen metabolism remains abnormal, as reflected in the ratio of plasma amino acids. Thus, a protein-free diet may reduce blood ammonia levels and be beneficial in improving signs of hepatic encephalopathy but does not correct amino acid imbalances.

Protein restriction can worsen other problems by causing low plasma protein concentrations to decrease further. Dietary effects on hepatic protein synthesis can be evaluated by plasma protein measurements. Hepatic metabolic functions require protein to support their structures. Dietary protein restriction compromises the liver's ability to synthesize proteins.

Protein restriction is indicated only with unmanageable hepatic encephalopathy. In other cases, dietary protein is not restricted but is adjusted to meet needs for synthesizing proteins and to prevent signs of hepatic encephalopathy, which, except in the acute case, may be of lesser importance. If possible, protein intake should be maintained at a minimum of one gram per 20 calories of food intake.

Protein Source

The source of protein is important to survival and affects the clinical signs of hepatic insufficiency. Dogs with experimentally produced disease and fed commercial dog food developed signs of hepatic encephalopathy and died within two to three months. Dogs with similar diseases and fed diets with protein from milk or soybeans developed no clinical signs and survived many months.[3,4] This study is similar to others showing survival time and clinical signs to be worse when meat rather than milk protein is fed.

At one time it was believed that survival is due to improved metabolism of branched-chain, aromatic, and sulfur-containing amino acids. However, abnormalities persist in amino acid metabolism on any diet. Moreover, when amino acid abnormalities are worsened by feeding excess aromatic amino acids, clinical signs do not worsen. Also, milk and soybean proteins have sulfur-containing amino acid contents similar to meat proteins in commercial dog foods. Milk protein and soybean protein diets could have lower ammoniagenic amino acids, such as threonine, glycine, serine, histidine, tryptophan, and lysine, but meat proteins have similar amounts of these amino acids.

Glutamine and glutamic acid comprise up to 20 percent of protein amino acid nitrogen. Following absorption, a high percentage of glutamine is converted to glutamate, releasing ammonia that represents one-half of portal blood ammonia. Controlling glutamine intake may benefit dogs and cats with hepatic insufficiency, but the glutamine-glutamate content of milk protein is relatively high, which suggests that glutamine is unimportant.

A number of other suggestions have been made to explain the beneficial effects of milk or soybean protein diets. The most important may be that a high ratio of carbohydrate to protein is essential in order to see a benefit.

The diet should contain minimum methionine. Excess methionine escapes intestinal absorption and enters the colon, where bacteria change it to a toxin. Absorption of this toxin worsens brain abnormalities seen with hepatic disease. Methionine-rich foods should be avoided.

Sometimes other amino acids are helpful in reducing signs of hepatic disease. Arginine and citrulline are two that directly or indirectly accelerate conversion of ammonia to urea. This can reduce ammonia's toxic effects on brain function. Proteins fed should contain high levels of these amino acids.

Hyperammonemia can also be managed with anything that causes frequent evacuation of colonic contents. Cathartics are sometimes used. Lactulose, an indigestible carbohydrate that ferments in the colon, is sometimes recommended. A more natural means of keeping the colon relatively empty is by feeding a natural source of starch that is poorly digested. Raw potato starch is poorly digested, and amounts exceeding what a dog or a cat will tolerate, greater than eight grams per kilogram body weight, will cause the feces to loosen, and evacuations will be more frequent.

■ Fats

Dietary fat is necessary as a source of calories and essential fatty acids; it also enhances palatability. A number of studies have shown that dogs and cats with hepatic disease (even cats with hepatic lipidosis) do well on diets containing 20 percent to 25 percent fat. In contrast to this tolerance of triglycerides, free fatty acids interfere with ammonia metabolism and contribute to hyperammonemia. They also contribute directly to hepatic encephalopathy. Most dietary fat is resynthesized into triglycerides and formed into chylomicrons before leaving intestinal epithelial cells. Thus, dietary fat does not increase plasma free fatty acids. Plasma free fatty acids increase during fasting when adipose triglycerides are catabolized for energy.

■ Vitamins and Minerals

Some nutrients can worsen liver damage. Vitamin A can be hepatotoxic. A small excess of vitamin A can act synergistically with other substances to damage the liver. For example, moderate levels of copper, iron, and many drugs are not toxic to the liver, but with a background of high but seemingly safe levels of vitamin A, the addition of one of these other substances can damage the liver. Also, endotoxin absorbed from the intestine normally has little effect on the liver. The addition of vitamin A, however, can act synergistically with the endotoxin to damage the liver. Therefore, supplementation to give excess vitamin A is not innocuous and can contribute to liver damage due to other causes.

The liver stores copper and has the highest concentration in the body. Copper is 10 times higher in a dog's liver than in a human's. That is not necessarily a species difference. More than likely the difference reflects the amount of copper consumed, being much greater in the dog. Before dogs ate commercial pet food, the content of copper in their livers was much lower than it is today. Figure 18.1 shows that the hepatic concentration of copper increased during the last 50 years from less than 10 micrograms copper per gram dry weight of liver to over 200 today. That 20-fold increase most likely resulted from a dietary level of copper in commercial pet foods that is much higher than needed.

Copper levels in pet food are important because copper can be toxic and cause both acute and chronic hepatic disease.[7,8] Chronic toxicity is

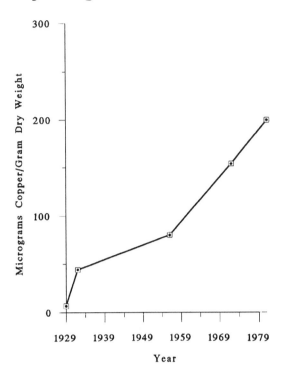

Figure 18.1. The concentration of copper in the livers of dogs over a 50-year period (adapted from Su et al., 1982).

frequent in dogs. The liver normally excretes copper in bile. Hepatic disease reduces excretion of copper in bile so that hepatic copper levels increase. Greater copper levels damage the liver further and worsen its ability to excrete copper. It is likely that the increasing hepatic copper concentrations in pet foods act with other insults to damage the liver and cause hepatic disease to be more common today. Dietary copper should be minimal with hepatic disease.

Many animals with hepatic disease are deficient in zinc. Zinc salts can be given to replace the deficit. Zinc is also useful because it competes with copper for intestinal absorption. Zinc supplements reduce copper absorption.

Vitamins E and K are useful with hepatic disease. Vitamin E protects against lipid peroxidation in cell membranes. Vitamin K is essential for normal blood clotting, which is often abnormal with hepatic disease.

Dogs make ascorbic acid in the liver, and it can be deficient with hepatic disease. With hepatic insufficiency plasma ascorbic acid can be lower than normal even when the patient is given recommended additions of a standard vitamin-mineral supplement. Ascorbic acid is also useful in protecting against liver damage. As an antioxidant it protects against lipid peroxidation.

■ Pet Food Contaminants

The diet should contain only minimal amounts of endotoxin and be free of chemicals. Diets prepared from wholesome foods accomplish that. As mentioned earlier, commercial pet foods can be high in endotoxin. Small amounts of endotoxin damage the liver. Very small amounts are usually not harmful unless other chemicals interact with the endotoxin to cause damage. Often these chemicals alone cause no hepatic damage.

Management with Drugs

Very few drugs are needed to treat hepatic disease. If possible, all drugs should be discontinued. Many drugs can damage the liver, and many others require hepatic conversion for their excretion. Hepatic drug conversion requires energy and nutrients that are needed for recovery of hepatic damage.

Chronic hepatic inflammation (hepatitis) requires corticosteroid treatment; inflammation persists without such treatment.[9] Cortisone causes hepatic degeneration that is not serious or life threatening, however. Thus, when inflammation disappears, corticosteroids are discontinued, and any drug damage disappears. Corticosteroids are not given when there is no hepatic inflammation.

Antibiotics are often useful for managing animals with hepatic disease. Drugs selected should not require metabolism by the liver. Such drugs include penicillins and aminoglycosides.

Other drugs are sometimes used for treating hepatic disease in humans. However, no other drugs are proven beneficial for hepatic disease in dogs and cats.

Diet Formulation for Dogs

A diet containing cottage cheese or tofu and a readily digested starch such as polished rice meets the nutritional requirements of dogs with hepatic disease. Fats, preferably animal, are added to enhance palatability and to provide essential fatty acids, and if the diet cannot be completely balanced, additional vitamins and minerals are given. Vitamin B$_{12}$ should be given by tablet several times a month or by feeding a food such as sardines that contains abundant amounts. Meat is not recommended since hepatic encephalopathy and shortened survival times may result when dogs with hepatic insufficiency are fed meat-based diets. Supplementation with mixtures of branched-chain amino acids offer no proven benefit. The protein content of the diet can be as low as 10 percent on a dry basis but should be increased with evidence of protein deficiency, such as hypoalbuminemia.

Diets for hepatic disease are balanced as necessary with vitamins and minerals. Requirements for B vitamins are determined by caloric intake. With complete anorexia there is no requirement; with resumption of food intake after a period of anorexia, there is a greater-than-maintenance need for these vitamins. Such animals should receive a doubled dose of water-soluble vitamins each day. Vitamin C supplementation may be necessary even when feeding a diet containing standard amounts of ascorbic acid. Ascorbic acid can be given up to 25 milligrams/kilogram body weight per day. Ascorbic acid can cause release of stored hepatic copper, and that can worsen hepatic pathology. Vitamin E can be given at levels of 500 milligrams/day to dogs and 100 milligrams/day to cats. Vitamin A is not given because it can interact synergistically with chemicals and toxins such as endotoxin to injure the liver. That happens with levels of vitamin A that are normally not hepatotoxic. Mineral supplementation can include zinc (3 mg/kilogram per day of zinc gluconate or 2 mg/kg/day zinc sulfate, each divided into three doses; zinc acetate (2 mg/kg/day) may be tolerated better with less chance of gastrointestinal irritation), based on studies that zinc inhibits intestinal copper absorption and its deposition in the liver. Hepatic copper accumulates in some dogs with hepatic disease, and high hepatic copper is toxic. The owner-prepared diets in this chapter are low in copper. If a low-copper intake is desired, supplements containing copper are not given. Dogs with hepatic disease causing copper retention should also not be fed commercial dog foods. They contain 5 to 10 mg copper/kg, as recommended by the National Research Council.

Diet Formulation for Cats

Cats must be fed a relatively high-protein diet. They are fed a balanced diet providing 80 to 100 kilocalories/kilogram body weight per day. Protein amounts should provide 12 to 20 percent of caloric needs, which is roughly twice that needed by dogs. There is little information on feeding cats with hepatic insufficiency. They are probably similar to other mammals in that feeding meat-protein diets worsens clinical signs and progression of hepatic pathology. However, it is difficult to find cats that accept meat-free diets, especially when they are anorectic due to hepatic disease. Diets containing milk or soybean protein offer little advantage because of their amino acid composition.

Although nonmeat diets may be beneficial because they include only small amounts of sulfur-containing amino acids, which can produce toxins, they are deficient in taurine, whose chronic lack can result in ocular and cardiac problems. Milk has little taurine, and vegetable proteins have essentially none, so a diet based on these proteins must be supplemented with 50 milligrams taurine per day for an adult cat. That can be provided by supplementing the diet with clams, which have taurine amounts that are up to seven times greater than for fish, beef, or chicken. Meat-protein-restricted diets can also be prepared.

Because most hepatic pathology is secondary to primary disease in nonhepatic tissue, dietary management is supportive or directed at the primary problem. In either case cats are fed 80 to 100 kilocalories/kilogram body weight per day, and 12 percent to 20 percent of their caloric needs must be provided by protein. In addition to taurine the diet must also contain adequate amounts of arginine.

An anorectic cat should be managed by feeding an enteral diet via a nasogastric or gastrostomy tube. A liquid enteral diet can be given slowly, which minimizes the possibility of vomiting or diarrhea often seen with enteral diets. Tube feeding eliminates a need for benzodiazepines or anabolic steroids to stimulate appetite. These drugs, like many, have side effects that are unwanted with hepatic disease.

The enteral diets are ideal because they are meat-free, being formulated from milk and soybean proteins. Most of these diets are high in fat, approximating 30 percent or more. There may be theoretical reasons for a high-fat diet contributing to hepatic encephalopathy, but that result is not seen. If most of the dietary calories are provided by carbohydrates, large volumes of enteral diets would be required. Enteral diets based on milk and soybean proteins require taurine supplementation: 150 milligrams is added to eight ounces of diet. Supplementation with branched-chain amino acids is of no benefit.

Owner-prepared diets can be used for cats with hepatic disease. Such diets are similar to ones prepared for dogs, but they need more protein and taurine. No commercial diets are produced for cats with hepatic disease. In general, many species of animals with hepatic insufficiency do more poorly and their pathology worsens when they are fed commercially prepared animal foods. Feeding such diets is probably unimportant for most cats with hepatic pathology, but any commercial diet is likely to be less effective than an enteral diet in a cat with serious hepatic disease.

Diets for cats should be supplemented with B vitamins, especially thiamine, because cats become deficient quite soon during anorexia. Recommendations for supplementation with fat-soluble vitamins is the same as for dogs. No recommendations can be given for supplementation with ascorbic acid and zinc because nothing is known about requirements for cats with hepatic disease.

Feeding Frequency for Dogs and Cats

Small meals are fed often to minimize hepatic encephalopathy caused by excess ammonia formed from glutamine metabolism and from excess protein entering the colon. Large single daily feedings of protein that exceed nitrogen needs are catabolized for energy or converted to triglycerides. Following deamination of proteins, additional ammonia must be converted to urea. Frequent feedings also reduce the time during which body protein is catabolized for energy. During fasting, muscle protein is catabolized to amino acids, which are deaminated and converted to glucose, and peripheral triglycerides are catabolized to free fatty acids, which are metabolized to ketone bodies for energy. Protein catabolism produces additional ammonia and perpetuates amino acid imbalances. The branched-chain amino acids and alanine are used primarily for energy, whereas the aromatic amino acids are metabolized in the liver and their rate of utilization is reduced with hepatic disease.

The potential toxic effects of free fatty acids appear during fasting, the time when their levels are highest. Long chain fatty acids are incompletely oxidized in the liver, forming octanoic acid, which contributes to encephalopathy.

Frequent feedings also benefit carbohydrate metabolism. Dogs with portasystemic shunts can have low normal blood glucose. Hypoglycemia, manifested during fasting, is due to reduced glucose availability and is prevented by frequent feedings. Since oral glucose tolerance is impaired in dogs with shunts, frequent feedings maintain above-normal glucose levels. However, the derangement is not severe enough to produce significant hyperglycemia.

Dietary Management of Dogs with Shunts

Dietary management of dogs with portasystemic shunts is not a successful long-term treatment; most of these dogs do not have normal life expectancies. Liver function deteriorates because of progressive hepatic atrophy. Clinical signs of depression often persist despite optimum dietary management. The long-term prognosis is poor for animals managed with controlled diets. Nonsurgical management of dogs with portasystemic shunts results in at least two-thirds dying or being euthanized. Of the remainder, 7 percent survive and do well on medical management; the outcome of the rest is unknown.

Diets for Dogs with Hepatic Disease

Cottage Cheese, Tofu, and Rice Diet (Moderate sodium)

½ cup cottage cheese, 1 percent fat

⅔ cup tofu, raw firm

1½ cups rice, long-grain, cooked

1 tablespoon chicken fat

¼ teaspoon salt substitute—potassium chloride

3 bonemeal tablets (10-grain or equivalent)

1 multiple vitamin tablet

Provides 651 calories, 36.9 grams protein, 21.8 grams fat, 0.280 percent sodium

Supports caloric needs of a 20-pound dog

Two to 3 ounces or more of raw potato (23 kilocalories/ounce) can be added to increase bowel movement frequency.

Cottage Cheese and Rice Diet (High-sodium)

1½ cups rice, long-grain, cooked

1 cup cottage cheese, 1 percent fat

1 tablespoon chicken fat

¼ teaspoon salt substitute—potassium chloride

3 bonemeal tablets (10-grain or equivalent)

1 multiple vitamin tablet

Provides 598 calories, 34.5 grams protein, 17.1 grams fat, 0.647 percent sodium

Supports caloric needs of an 18-pound dog

Two to 3 ounces or more of raw potato (23 kilocalories/ounce) can be used to increase bowel movement frequency.

Tofu and Rice Diet (Low-sodium)

1⅓ cup tofu, raw firm

1½ cups rice, long-grain, cooked

2 teaspoons chicken fat

¼ teaspoon salt substitute—potassium chloride

3 bonemeal tablets (10-grain or equivalent)

1 multiple vitamin tablet

Provides 700 calories, 43.1 grams protein, 24.1 grams fat, 0.012 percent sodium

Supports caloric needs of a 22-pound dog

Two to 3 ounces or more of raw potato (23 kilocalories/ounce) can be used to increase bowel movement frequency.

Diets for Cats with Hepatic Disease

Cottage Cheese, Tofu, and Rice Diet (*Moderate sodium*)

½ cup cottage cheese, 1 percent fat

⅔ cup tofu, raw firm

⅓ cup rice, long-grain, cooked

1 ounce clams, chopped in juice

1 tablespoon chicken fat

2 bonemeal tablets (10-grain or equivalent)

1 multiple vitamin tablet

Provides 466 calories, 40.9 grams protein, 22.6 grams fat, 0.416 percent sodium

A 10-pound cat needs 318 calories per day (286 calories for a 9-pound and 350 calories for an 11-pound cat).

One to 2 ounces or more of raw potato (23 kilocalories/ ounce) can be used to increase bowel movement frequency.

Tofu and Rice Diet (*Low-sodium*)

1 cup tofu, raw firm

⅓ cup rice, long-grain, cooked

1 ounce clams, chopped in juice

1 tablespoon chicken fat

2 bonemeal tablets (10-grain or equivalent)

1 multiple vitamin tablet

Provides 463 calories, 36.3 grams protein, 25 grams fat, 0.036 percent sodium

A 10-pound cat needs 318 calories per day (286 calories for a 9-pound and 350 calories for an 11-pound cat).

One to 2 ounces or more of raw potato (23 kilocalories/ ounce) can be used to increase bowel movement frequency.

Turkey and Rice Diet (Low- to moderate sodium)

⅓ pound turkey (raw weight), cooked

⅓ cup rice, long-grain, cooked

2 bonemeal tablets (10-grain or equivalent)

1 multiple vitamin tablet

Provides 321 calories, 28.3 grams protein, 15.4 grams fat, 0.133 percent sodium

A 10-pound cat needs 318 calories per day (286 calories for a 9-pound and 350 calories for an 11-pound cat).

One to 2 ounces or more of raw potato (23 kilocalories/ ounce) can be used to increase bowel movement frequency.

References

1. Guilford, W. Grant. 1996. Approach to clinical problems in gastroenterology. In *Strombeck's Small Animal Gastroenterology*, edited by W. Grant Guilford, Sharon A. Center, Donald R. Strombeck, David A. Williams, and Denny J. Meyer, 50–76. Philadelphia: W.B. Saunders.

2. Rutgers, H.C. Carolien and John G. Harte. 1994. Hepatic disease. In *The Waltham Book of Clinical Nutrition of the Dog and Cat*, edited by J.M. Wills and K.W. Simpson, 239–276. Oxford: Pergamon Press.

3. Marks, Stanley L., Quinton R. Rogers, and Donald R. Strombeck. 1994. Nutritional support in hepatic disease. Part I. Metabolic alterations and nutritional considerations in dogs and cats. *Compendium Continuing Education Practicing Veterinarians*, 16:971–979.

4. Marks, Stanley L., Quinton R. Rogers, and Donald R. Strombeck. 1994. Nutritional support in hepatic disease. Part II. Dietary management of common liver disorders in dogs and cats. *Compendium Continuing Education Practicing Veterinarians*, 16:1287–1296.

5. Guilford, W. Grant. 1996. Nutritional management of gastrointestinal diseases. In *Strombeck's Small Animal Gastroenterology*, edited by W. Grant Guilford, Sharon A. Center, Donald R. Strombeck, David A. Williams, and Denny J. Meyer, 889–910. Philadelphia: W.B. Saunders.

6. Biourge, Vincent, Paul Pion, Julia Lewis, James G. Morris, and Quinton R. Rogers. 1993. Spontaneous occurrence of hepatic lipidosis in a group of laboratory cats. *Journal of Veterinary Internal Medicine* 7:194–197.

7. Twedt, David C., Irmin Sternlieb, and Steven R. Gilbertson. 1979.

Clinical, morphologic, and chemical studies on copper toxicosis of Bedlington terriers. *Journal of the American Veterinary Medical Association* 175:269–275.

8. Su, Le-Chu, Charles A. Owen, Paul E. Zollman and Robert Hardy, 1982. *American Journal of Physiology* 243 (Gastrointestinal Liver Physiology 6) G231-G236.

9. Center, Sharon A. 1996. Chronic hepatitis, cirrhosis, breed-specific hepatopathies, copper storage hepatopathy, suppurative hepatitis, granulomatous hepatitis, and idiopathic hepatic fibrosis. In *Strombeck's Small Animal Gastroenterology*, edited by W. Grant Guilford, Sharon A. Center, Donald R. Strombeck, David A. Williams, and Denny J. Meyer, 705–765. Philadelphia: W.B. Saunders.

INDEX